Also by Angelo Acquista, M.D.

THE SURVIVAL GUIDE

The Mediterranean Prescription

The Mediterranean Prescription

Meal Plans and Recipes
to Help You Stay Slim and Healthy
for the Rest of Your Life

Angelo Acquista, M.D.,
with Laurie Anne Vandermolen

Ballantine Books / New York

No book can replace the diagnostic expertise and medical advice of a trusted physician. Please be certain to consult with your doctor before making any decisions that affect your health, particularly if you suffer from any medical condition or have any symptom that may require treatment.

Published in the United States by Ballantine Books, an imprint of The Random House Publishing Group, a division of Random House, Inc., New York.

BALLANTINE and colophon are registered trademarks of Random House, Inc.

Library of Congress Cataloging-in-Publication Data

Acquista, Angelo.
The Mediterranean prescription : meal plans and recipes to help you stay slim and healthy for the rest of your life / by Angelo Acquista with Laurie Anne Vandermolen.
p. cm.
Includes index.
ISBN 0-345-47924-6
1. Nutrition. 2. Diet—Mediterranean Region. 3. Cookery, Mediterranean.
I. Vandermolen, Laurie Anne. II. Title.

RA784.A257 2006
613.2—dc22
2005044489

Printed in the United States of America on acid-free paper

www.ballantinebooks.com

4 6 8 9 7 5

Book design by Susan Turner

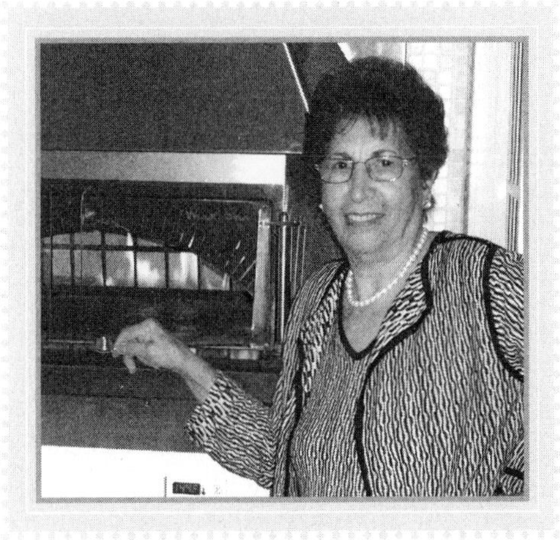

To my mother, Sara Acquista

Acknowledgments

Much of what I have accomplished in cooking has been through the somewhat painful trials and tribulations of trying, failing, and finally succeeding. During the many times it takes to get a recipe exactly right, my family has always been there to offer advice, help with preparation, and taste test the new creation. Most important, they have been there to inspire me to cook in the first place. My mother, Rosaria "Sara" Acquista, especially, passed on her interest in cooking to me. This passion caught up others as well, as the rest of my family, including my brother and his wife, Dominick and Cathy Acquista, and even their three children—Salvatore, Dominick, and Sara—have picked up the family tradition. My father has always supported my efforts, and in recent years has joined me in the kitchen as well. My dear friends Dr. V. A. Subramanian and William Hyman have also tried all of the new recipes—enduring the bad ones and helping guide me to the good ones.

I am also indebted to the late Dr. Peter Saita, who was not only my mentor and inspiration to become a doctor, but who also devised the original diet plan I use that has changed the lives of so many of my patients.

I am tremendously grateful to my medical writer, Laurie Vandermolen, who expertly researched and shaped this book and made my vision a reality.

This book would not have been possible without the efforts of many people: Danielle Durkin, my most excellent editor at Ballantine; Laura Dail, my first-rate agent; and Michael Feldman, coordinator extraordinaire. I would like them to know how appreciative I was of their understanding while my father was ill, and I thank them all for helping me pursue this project.

Thank you also to my nephews Angelo Acquista, for helping prepare many of the recipes, and Dominick Acquista, for aiding with the preliminary research; to Susan Raatz, Ph.D., R.D., for her expert nutritional advice and dedication to accuracy; and to Rachel Dugas and Brigid-Ann Dibella, for their support in preparing the manuscript.

Laurie Vandermolen would like to thank Danielle Durkin for her perpetual enthusiasm, patience, wisdom, and good cheer; as well as Michael Feldman, for expertly managing this project with finesse and humor; Laura Dail, for her inspiration and dedication; Dr. Raatz, for her invaluable expertise and assistance; and, of course, Dr. Acquista, for giving her the opportunity and privilege to write for him. She also wishes to extend her never-ending gratitude to her friends and family—especially Mom, Dad, Julie, Sheryl, Alex, Charlie, Levi, Brendan, Peter, Joe, Brian, Mary Ball, and most of all Bob—*her* prescription for life.

Contents

The Mediterranean Prescription

1

The Mediterranean Prescription

When I was a young college student in New York, my father introduced me to a wise, older doctor named Dr. Peter Saita. He was a Sicilian internist who practiced in downtown Manhattan and over time became somewhat of a mentor to me. He used to tell me that being a doctor was the noblest profession, and it was he who inspired me to go to medical school. I kept up my relationship with him throughout medical school and would often accompany him to see patients. He would tell me, "The best thing I can do for my patients is to get them to stop smoking and to help them lose weight." This was in the 1970s, when people didn't really pay attention to these issues. He personally saw the connection between being overweight and poor health among his patients and took it upon himself to help those at risk. As a result, he developed a diet that he would describe briefly to his overweight patients, so easy to follow that he didn't even have to write it down, that he saw work over and over. He handed this down to me, a newly graduated doctor, and I never forgot it—in part because I had so much respect for this man, but mostly because, as I eventually found again and again with my own patients, *it worked.*

Years ago as I was starting out as a physician, I tried to help patients lose weight in a more traditional way. I used to tell them how to eat healthily, would give them papers on nutrition, and would refer them to nutritionists, but they weren't losing weight. In my frustration, I tried telling them about Dr. Saita's diet. I said, "Why don't you try this very simple diet?" They would come back to me for a follow-up telling me, "I tried the diet, but it's difficult. I can't stick to it." I noticed that my American patients didn't have the devotion to food that was found in the Italian culture I grew up in. When I told them the diet included all-you-can-eat fish and chicken entrées, they thought fish had to mean salmon or tuna, when there are so many kinds of fish out there. They also didn't know how to cook it, nor did they have healthy, flavorful recipes for chicken. So I took the time to help them lose weight by writing recipes down on my prescription pad to get them started. I would say, "Look, it's not hard. You just have to be creative. Here, try these," and I'd scribble a couple of fish or chicken recipes down for them, based on my and my mother's Sicilian recipes. And miraculously, my patients started losing weight. They couldn't believe the easy and delicious meals they could eat while they were losing weight.

Initially, I would prescribe the diet to patients who had illnesses that had clear connections to being overweight, such as hypertension, type 2 diabetes (as opposed to type 1, which you're born with), and sleep apnea. As my medical practice continued, however, it became apparent how much being overweight set the stage for untold numbers of illnesses and diseases, and how important it was to lose weight as *preventive* medicine.

My patient profile is no different from the patient population of doctors' offices around the country. My new patients are coming in increasingly heavier, and the illnesses related to being overweight and obese are becoming much more frequent. The weight of Americans has been rising at an astonishing rate since the early 1960s due to a combination of diet, meal size, activity habits, genetics, and food industry and media influence. As most people know by now, either by reading statistics or by just glancing around themselves at a crowded location, around *two-thirds* of our citizens are either overweight or obese. And there appears to be every indication that this trend will continue. Not coincidentally, the United States is in the midst of major epidemics of heart disease, stroke, high blood pressure, cancer, type 2 diabetes, and hepatitis. These conditions are all clearly exacerbated, if not caused, by excess weight and are major causes of disability and death in this nation. They also account for a significant amount of our health care dollars.

THE SHOCKING STATISTICS

- Approximately two out of three Americans are either overweight or obese (compared with fewer than one out of four in the early 1960s); around 127 million American adults are overweight, with 44–60 million of them obese, and 9 million severely obese.
- Approximately 15 percent of children ages six to nineteen are overweight or obese; this prevalence has nearly tripled in the past three decades.
- Obesity may shorten life span by five to twenty years.
- Obesity is currently associated with greater disease and poorer health-related quality of life than smoking, problem drinking, and poverty.
- The World Bank has estimated the cost of obesity in the United States at 12 percent of the national health care budget, according to the Worldwatch Institute.
- The leading causes of death in the United States are all exacerbated or caused by excess weight.
    - Heart disease is the leading cause of death in the United States.
    - Cancer is the second-leading cause.
    - Stroke is the third-leading cause.
    - Type 2 diabetes (95 percent of diabetics) is currently the sixth-ranking cause of death, and it recently became the fourth-leading cause of death in New York City. Type 2 diabetes also increases the risk of heart attack and stroke by two to four times and is the leading cause of blindness, fatal kidney disease, and lower extremity amputations.

In addition to helping people look better and feel better, which I am all for, it's terribly important to reverse this trend of health problems in our country. People may be living longer due to advances in medication and health care management, but many diseases can be greatly improved or completely prevented without the use of drugs or surgical intervention. Take insulin resistance. Highly related to being overweight, it is a condition in which your body fails to respond properly to insulin. Around a fourth of Americans have it, unbeknownst to them, and it puts them at significant risk for developing full-blown diabetes. The first line of defense for this condition is—you guessed it—losing weight. Even a small percentage of weight loss can help appreciably. So, I am sure you want to know, how do you get there?

Let me tell you a little bit about the healthiest known diet in the world. In the 1950s, the role of diet in human health was a mystery. Most researchers accepted that there was a connection between diet and disease, but the nature of this connection was largely unstudied in human populations. In 1958, a young physician named Ancel Keys of the University of Minnesota, along with a team of international scientists, set out to understand one disease in particular, the disease that was killing more people around the world than any other: heart disease.

Animal studies had suggested that fats were to blame for heart disease, but there was only anecdotal evidence for humans. During World War II, for example, Keys had observed that heart disease rates plummeted in countries with shortages of meat and dairy products, both rich in saturated fats. In addition, when he and his wife had traveled around Europe and Africa measuring blood cholesterol levels in preliminary studies in the early 1950s, he noticed that affluent people, who were eating more meat and dairy products, had higher cholesterol and suffered more heart attacks than poorer people who could only afford limited amounts of those foods. Keys thus speculated that saturated fat might be the root of the problem and was responsible for increasing the risk of heart disease.

To test his hypothesis, Keys and his co-investigators looked at the diets, lifestyles, blood pressures, and blood cholesterol levels of more than twelve thousand healthy middle-aged men from Greece, Italy, Japan, Finland, the Netherlands, Yugoslavia, and the United States. For the first time, investigators were actually stationed in people's homes to monitor what they were eating and sending samples back to their own laboratory for analysis, rather than relying on food-intake questionnaires. They then followed up after five, ten, fifteen, and twenty years. It came to be known as the Seven Countries Study, one of the greatest and most influential epidemiological studies of our time.

Ten years after the study began, men from east Finland were faring the worst: 28 percent of them had developed heart disease. It turns out the Finns were eating more saturated fat than almost anyone in the world—24 percent of their calories. That's double what Americans eat now. The residents of the fishing villages that were studied in Japan ate the least fat overall and the least saturated fat. Only 5 percent of them developed heart disease—far better than the Finns. But it wasn't the best. That honor went to the men from the Greek island of Crete. After ten years, only 2 percent of them had developed heart disease, and none of them had died. Amazingly, the Cretans were eating about as much total fat as the artery-clogged Finns—30 to 40 percent of their total daily calories came from fat. The difference was that their intake of saturated fat was far lower. It was not, however, as low as that of the mostly rice-and-vegetables Japanese diet.

When the blood cholesterol of the Cretans was measured, they had the lowest levels of any group. This was a conundrum, because the investigators had been assuming that saturated fat from the diet played a principle role in one's blood cholesterol level. How could the Cretans—who ate more saturated fat than the Japanese—be healthier than the Japanese, who ate hardly any saturated fat? This mystery was answered when it was learned that the kinds of unsaturated fats they were eating were also making a difference. The Cretans were getting nearly half of their fat from olive oil, a monounsaturated fat, and it created the best lipid profile for a human body that you could ask for. Keys thus established one of the most important pieces of knowledge we can arm ourselves with for good health: by monitoring the *kinds* of fat we eat, more so than the amount, we can minimize or prevent heart disease, the number one worldwide killer.

The Seven Countries Study also determined that rates of death from all causes, age for age, were among the lowest in the Mediterranean regions. The Seven Countries Study was essentially the launch for many studies to follow over the next several decades to try to elucidate what makes the Mediterranean diet so healthy, in addition to dramatically reducing heart disease. Currently it appears that concentrating on fresh, unprocessed food that was largely plant-based—along with some fish, olive oil, dairy, wine, and a little red meat—gave people of the Mediterranean the magic formula. Their diet had the best combination of fats, was high in complex carbohydrates and fiber, and was also rich in a combination of antioxidants, phytochemicals, vitamins, and minerals—the total effect of which cannot be duplicated with pills or supplements. These investigations have also taught us that, in addition to heart disease, the Mediterranean diet can help prevent obesity, heart attacks, cancer, arthritis, type 2 diabetes, hypertension, and the metabolic syndrome, among others.

In reading about Keys's studies, I learned that his first destination, back in 1952, was the southern Italian town of Naples. He was drawn there because of the reports he'd heard that heart disease barely existed among Neapolitans. As it turned out, area doctors confirmed that their hospitals rarely had coronary patients; the only cases were seen at private clinics for the well-to-do. The men of the working class—who couldn't afford the meats and dairy the upper classes could—had remarkably low cholesterol and almost no heart trouble. But the thing that struck me most about his experience was when he described the simple yet irresistible cuisine of the region:

> The ordinary food of the common Neapolitans consisted of homemade minestrone/vegetable soup, pasta in endless variety, always freshly cooked, served with tomato sauce and a sprinkle of cheese, only occasionally enriched with some bits of meat, or served with a little local seafood without any cheese; a hearty dish of beans and macaroni; lots of whole-grain bread never more than a few hours from the oven and never served with any kind of spread; great quantities of fresh vegetables; a modest portion of meat or fish perhaps twice a week; red wine; always fresh fruit for dessert.

When Keys was asked years later to formulate a diet that might serve as a preventive against coronary heart disease, he could come up with nothing more suited for this purpose than the traditional working-class diet of early 1950s Naples. I realized with astonishment that he was talking about the diet I grew up on.

Sicily—an island off the southern coast of Italy and a place of dramatic beauty, history, and dazzlingly fresh and healthy cuisine—is the largest island in the Mediterranean. It's also the island I lived on until the age of nine, when my family moved to America. I lived in a small, hilly town near the Mediterranean Sea called Castrofilippo. To me it's the most beautiful place on earth—rugged, rocky, and colorful, with weather the most optimal in the world. Springtime occurs in February, and then there's virtually no rain from May to September. We had an abundance of different varieties of fruits and vegetables because of this climate. In fact, there were very few if any grocery stores where you'd buy vegetables because everyone grew their own. What's more, it was actually a necessity to eat a diet rich in vegetables, legumes, fruits, homemade whole-grain breads and pasta, and olive oil made from the olives of our own trees—even our wine was made from our own grapevines—because most people were poor and couldn't afford to buy much, meat in particular; meat was considered to be a luxury. However, because of our proximity to the ocean, we always had fresh fish available to us. Perhaps partly because of our limited access to a vast selection of foods, such as the options Americans have at their disposal today, we made the most of what we had and paid a lot of attention to food preparation, flavor, and mealtimes.

It should be noted, however, that though the culture I grew up in ate the traditional Mediterranean diet, it's not the case today. As my town as well as the rest of the Mediterranean became more affluent over the years, the diet of its inhabitants slowly became more Westernized, with more meats, dairy, and other sources of saturated fat entering into the diet, as well as refined grains. So even though the Mediterranean has historically been a healthy and lean region, it is not so anymore. Many more people there are carrying excess weight from their more Americanized diets—and American weight-related health problems have followed.

Because of the great benefits of the Mediterranean diet, I decided to adapt my weight-loss diet so that it could ease people into this exceptionally healthy way of eating. My goal was to take people from a rapid weight-loss phase with Mediterranean-style recipes into a maintenance plan in which they will be fully "eating Mediterranean." I designed it so that in the first two weeks you should lose five to ten pounds if you follow the diet plan closely. For those who wish to lose more than that, they can continue on the Two-Week Weight Loss Stage. When you are ready, you can transition to the Maintenance Stage. I knew the plan had to be practical, livable, effortless, and most of all delicious, or no one would adopt it into their lives. Once I had the foundation, I took it upon myself to select the perfect recipes for the plan.

While I come from a family with a long tradition of cooking, I never cooked until I went to medical school. It began as a matter of necessity. The deal I had with my roommates was that I would cook and they would wash the dishes. They soon caught on that I was getting my mother to make the meatballs and sauce. I would heat up some pasta, throw the premade meatballs and sauce over the pasta, and then go into my bedroom to relax. My roommates were faintly annoyed, but they couldn't resist the meals, so they let me continue for the whole first year of school. As time wore on, though, in the second and third years of medical school, I'd call my mother to get advice on how she made this or that. I began to keep her on the phone with me the whole time I was cooking. It was fun for me to cook and for us to bond in this way. And my roommates continued to do all the cleaning. At this point, they were so supportive of the deal that they started coming home early so we could all eat together.

Eventually I began cooking for family and countless friends as well, and it became a big part of my life. I love making and creating delicious dishes and then sharing them. Trying my recipes definitely seems to be my patients' favorite part of my diet. It makes me feel great that they enjoy them so much and that they are taking pleasure in something I provided. In fact, it's no surprise that the Mediterranean diet has demonstrated over and over in studies that because of its palatability, people are able to stick with it, much more so than other diets. You can eat Chicken Cacciatore, Grilled Shrimp with Thyme, Sweet-and-Sour Red Snapper, Halibut N.S.E.W. (potato halibut), Striped Bass Oreganato, Lentil Soup, and Pasta with Peas, Asparagus, and Tomato Sauce—now, that doesn't sound like deprivation, does it?

I want to emphasize that it's not just about the food, however. Part of the wonderful beneficial health effects from living in the Mediterranean just may be due to the lifestyle as well. During the postwar era, when the studies were done, Mediterraneans were physically active, had a slower pace of living, relied on and communed with family and friends, and—probably as a result of all of the above—had less stress. They had great reverence for the food on their table. I greatly encourage you to follow their course. Take the time to eat. Take the time to do what's important in life, which is to make good food and share it with friends and family. These meals are highly nutritious for the whole family (anyone over the age of two), so prepare them to share. I truly believe this is one of the problems our country faces—we have deemphasized dinnertime with our families and the importance of food in our daily lives.

Mealtime should be a time to enjoy, gather, savor, and linger. Food should be a pleasure, not a forbidden, dreaded part of life ridden with anxiety and guilt. I have created delicious, easy-to-follow recipes as a starting point. My goal in helping you make a lasting change in weight and health was to make a plan that was desirable, pleasurable, simple, and maintainable, and I think I have done that. It cannot be a regimented, day-by-day rule book; it must be infinitely variable and flexible, able to adjust to a person's cravings and degree of hunger, the contents of the refrigerator, or the offerings at whatever restaurant he or she winds up at. Moreover, in place of food that is mouth-watering and high in calories, there must be something healthy but equally mouth-watering and easy to attain, and that is what this book provides.

You can change your life if you follow my plan. You need to be at your best weight to be your best self, and I want to help you get there. In essence, when you become fit, you become able to free your mind from worrying about weight control and instead can concentrate on the things that matter most to you in life. First and foremost, you need to get rid of the idea of "keeping it off." I think most people who feel they have excess pounds feel "overweight"—that is, like a normal-size person who is over his or her natural weight. "Keeping it off" implies you are a fat person struggling to maintain an unnaturally thin state. Instead, I will show you how to find your comfortable weight and stay there. Once you've reached your new set point, the reduction of your cravings and your new mind-set will make you feel as if you belong there, not that you're fighting anything. The struggle is over. This book is not just a quick fix for the high school reunion; it's a prescription for life.

SUCCESS STORIES

TED: LOST 95 POUNDS OVER 8 MONTHS

I had gained quite a bit of weight after a debilitating injury that caused me to be extremely sedentary for quite a while. Dr. Acquista put me on his diet and wrote out a bunch of recipes for me on his prescription pad. It's the best diet I've ever been on, bar none. I thought the recipes were very tasty and very satisfying. I think that was a big key for me. It really helped me to have a dinner where I could eat as much as I wanted, because it made me feel a little like I was cheating. It wasn't about portion control, such an awful part of other diets. This doesn't feel like a diet; it feels like I've been to a restaurant and had a wonderful, gourmet meal.

The first few weeks I struggled a little with cravings, but it was okay since I was just starting out and was highly motivated, so I could ignore them. I added a few things back in, like some fruit, whole-grain bread, 2 percent milk, low-fat yogurt, sugar-free sorbet, and some pasta. Personally, I try to keep the olive oil down somewhat because of all the calories. Anyway, working out really helped with the cravings, because it made me feel like I'm putting so much into this, I'm not going to ruin it by going out and eating double hamburgers and ice cream. The cravings really stopped once I started exercising.

What I find most amazing was the relatively short duration required for a dramatic weight loss. Other plans would say it would take a couple of years of being disciplined, and I didn't feel I could wait that long. Once the weight comes off, you can eat a much more varied diet and can exercise less to maintain your weight.

My health also improved on the diet. I'd been suffering from sleep apnea, which improved greatly, while fatigue, elevated liver test results, and high blood pressure totally disappeared.

MARTI: LOST 15 POUNDS ON THE TWO-WEEK WEIGHT LOSS STAGE

I have been trying to lose weight for a couple of years. I lost weight before but had to do it without eating things I liked, so after I went off the diet, I inevitably gained the weight back. I loved this diet because I could eat foods I like and I still lost weight. Also, I didn't eat any red meat for two weeks and my digestion got so much better. I have much more energy now and also think that my skin looks better.

ROB: LOST 10 POUNDS ON THE TWO-WEEK WEIGHT LOSS STAGE

My wife and I really enjoyed cooking and eating the dinner options together. As opposed to previous diets I've done, which made me feel deprived, I felt like the Mediterranean Prescription left me feeling sated. I was especially impressed with the results, given that a recent knee injury had curtailed my physical activity. Thanks, Dr. Acquista!

CHARLES: LOST 46 POUNDS OVER 8 MONTHS

I didn't do the rapid weight-loss program but went straight to the maintenance stage because I wanted more variety in my daily meals than what the diet plan offered. My meals were often fish, pasta in moderation, and two vegetables, maybe five times a week. I had red meat about once a week. I ate a lot of fruits and nuts. The weight started coming off and it did not feel like dieting whatsoever. I always felt full. Prior to the weight loss I had daily fatigue and was falling asleep at the wheel of my car. I also had high blood pressure. These conditions have both resolved. My blood pressure is back to normal, so my blood pressure medication has been reduced to half; if it stays this way for another month, I'll come off the medication completely.

SHEREE: LOST 6 POUNDS ON THE TWO-WEEK WEIGHT LOSS STAGE

This is the most effective diet I've ever tried. Since I am not technically overweight, 6 pounds in two weeks (and I went off the diet twice) is a wonderful result for me. The meals were easy to prepare, and since it included all types of seafood, there was a lot of variety. I particularly enjoyed using olive oil and balsamic vinegar. I enjoyed the experience and will incorporate many of the meals into my regular diet. It's nice to know that if extra pounds creep on, I can go back to the Two-Week Stage and quickly get them off.

JERRY: LOST 19 POUNDS OVER 7 WEEKS

I lost 19 pounds without really trying. The diet was just very easy to stick to. The recipes were phenomenal, so I never got bored, which was a very nice part of Dr. Acquista's plan. There was no plain boiled chicken and things like that; there was something new every night. I ate out a lot as well but just stuck to the plan at restaurants. I wasn't exercising, and cheated a little with the occasional cocktail, but the weight came right off. I keep telling all my friends that they have to try this diet, I'm that excited about it.

THE PLAN

A WEIGHT LOSS DIET IS NOT GOING TO CHANGE YOUR LIFE. THIS MAY SOUND surprising coming from a doctor who is going to teach you how to lose weight, but I agree with the results of all of the largest studies on diets that have been done: most diets don't work for long-term weight loss. Even commercial weight loss programs have abysmal results. One of the few that have given themselves over to a published, controlled scientific study is Weight Watchers, and it reported only a 3 percent sustainable weight loss (that's like a 200-pound person losing 6 pounds). This amount of weight loss can have health benefits for some, depending on your body mass index (BMI), but it is probably far short of most people's goals. You probably know from your own experience that most diets don't work. Many people gain the weight right back, and often extra pounds on top of that.

In order to permanently change your weight, you must master three principles:

- Reduce your body fat, which will in turn reduce your appetite.
- Increase your physical activity.
- Change your eating habits.

There are a million claims out there, but in the scientific literature, these are three proven elements that will give you the ammunition to end your battle to maintain a healthy weight. It's not about timing, special food combinations, restricting food groups, or grapefruit. Brilliant scientists are in their labs around the world at this very moment studying weight loss—there is big money in it, after all—and they have yet to come to any universal agreement about what works except the basic principles listed above.

The first one is not as obvious as it may seem. As your body fat increases, so does your appetite. Fat cells aren't just receptacles, they're like little living, breathing survival machines. They send out signals to get you to eat more so they don't perish. They don't know how many other fat cells there are around them that will get you through the next famine, and they don't care that you'd prefer to wear a bikini this upcoming summer. While your appetite can increase initially when losing weight, losing fat will help control your appetite once you settle into your new set point: after a while post–weight loss, your shrunken fat cells will become less metabolically active, thus slowing down the signaling to your brain. Many of my patients will tell me that before they lost weight, they felt like food controlled them instead of the other way around. A box of cookies in the house meant a box of cookies eaten, possibly in one sitting. Once you get down below a certain threshold, however, your body fat is not screaming at you to save it anymore. Food doesn't control you; hunger is like a minor headache you can ignore if you want to. You could even keep a cupboard stocked with sweets, and they wouldn't be any more tempting to you than a head of broccoli. So you need a plan that is sustainable, that allows you to eat the foods you love (we're talking about a prescription for life here), that allows you to feel full, and that reduces fat tissue.

Increasing your physical activity will help ensure weight loss. High-speed weight-loss programs can get you to lose weight, but the early reduction in pounds comes primarily from losing water weight or muscle tissue, not weight from fat tissue. The initial weight loss from low-carbohydrate diets is water weight. By eating fewer carbohydrates, your body burns its stored carbohydrates (in the form of glycogen) for energy. When your body burns glycogen, water is released, so you lose weight. If you're losing weight too fast, you'll also be burning valuable, metabolic-rate-increasing muscle tissue. What you *want* to be doing, of course, is burning *fat*. Exercise compensates for this phenomenon by increasing muscle and burning fat. A multitude of studies shows that regular exercise also prevents weight regain.

People on diets are often looking for the quick fix and see a diet as a solution to a short-term problem. On the contrary, after weight loss, if you want to maintain a healthy weight, you need to adopt lifelong healthy habits. I have a friend who was on a diet and the whole time kept commenting that she couldn't wait to finish it so she could start eating Doritos again. Of course, she went right back to her former weight when she stopped the diet. But who wants to be on a diet for the rest of his or her life? My plan is to teach you healthy eating habits without sacrificing feeling utterly satisfied.

To achieve the three goals I have outlined above, I have devised a comprehensive plan with two basic stages: the **TWO-WEEK WEIGHT LOSS STAGE** and the **MAINTENANCE STAGE.**

The Two-Week Weight Loss Stage is designed to help you lose weight immediately, kick some bad eating habits, reduce your appetite, and maybe get you into your skinny jeans if you don't have that much to lose. If you haven't reached your target weight in two weeks, you may continue on this phase in order to drop pounds. True, the first program is technically a "diet," but this is only the beginning.

The Maintenance Stage is the most important part of the Mediterranean Prescription, because this is the part that's going to change your eating habits, change your life, and probably give you a few extra years. While other diet books focus on weight loss, this book also features what comes after. The Maintenance Stage is based on the Mediterranean diet, which allows you to effortlessly maintain your weight (preventing weight regain after the diet, and preventing the gradual creep upward on the scale that most people experience as they age) while helping your heart and helping prevent cancer and other chronic diseases. Since I'm from Sicily, my recipes have an Italian bent, but you can follow the principles of this book eating cuisine from any part of the Mediterranean region, such as Greece, Turkey, France, Spain, the Middle East, and North Africa. Some of my patients skip the two-week plan entirely and go directly to this stage, and by just changing their eating habits lose weight.

If you choose to begin with the Two-Week Weight Loss Stage, I highly recommend that you be strict on it; it is the most difficult leg of my plan, and it will help disrupt unhealthy eating practices such as a dependence on unhealthy fats and poor snacking habits. Move on to the Maintenance Stage when you are ready. In the event that you really get off track and want to lose some quick pounds to get back down, simply follow the Two-Week Weight Loss Stage again.

Finally, even if you don't want or need to lose any weight, incorporating some of the principles of the Mediterranean Prescription into your diet will make you a healthier person than you were before.

TWELVE GUIDING PRINCIPLES

The thing I can't stress enough to my patients is how simple the Mediterranean Prescription really is. It's composed of twelve guiding principles—just twelve elements that, when taken together, can help prevent obesity, heart disease, and cancer and add years to your life, as study after study has shown. Not to mention that it's rich in fiber, protein, and micronutrients that help satiate and suppress your appetite, so you never feel hungry. It allows for decadent meals (see the recipe section), so you never feel deprived. I've included information in the text on how each component helps keep you healthy and how it can contribute both to weight loss and to easily maintaining your weight once it's off. While Maintenance Stage eating is not designed for losing weight, some people—depending on their individual combination of weight, body type, age, gender, and level of physical activity—will lose weight if they use the Mediterranean Prescription's principles to change their unhealthy eating habits.

THE TWELVE GUIDING PRINCIPLES OF THE MEDITERRANEAN PRESCRIPTION

1. Eat lots of **fruits.**
2. Eat lots of **vegetables.**
3. Eat lots of **legumes** (such as beans, peas, and lentils).
4. Eat lots of **nuts and seeds.**
5. Eat lots of **whole grains,** especially whole-grain bread.
6. Use **olive oil** liberally, both in salads and in cooking.
7. Consume a moderate amount of **low-fat dairy products.**
8. Eat **fish.**
9. **Eat the right fats** (have a high ratio of unsaturated fats to saturated fats in your diet).
10. Engage in regular **physical activity.**
11. Drink **wine** (especially red) in moderation, if you choose.
12. Eat only small amounts of red meat and meat products.

The Mediterranean Prescription Pyramid

The following pyramid summarizes the daily, weekly, and monthly recommendations of the Mediterranean Prescription. Herein lies the heart of the plan. If you simply followed the proportions in this pyramid and read no further, you would be in fine shape and on your way to a healthier, fitter future. The recommendations shown here are for the Maintenance Stage. If you would like to lose weight, however, see Chapter 2 for guidance.

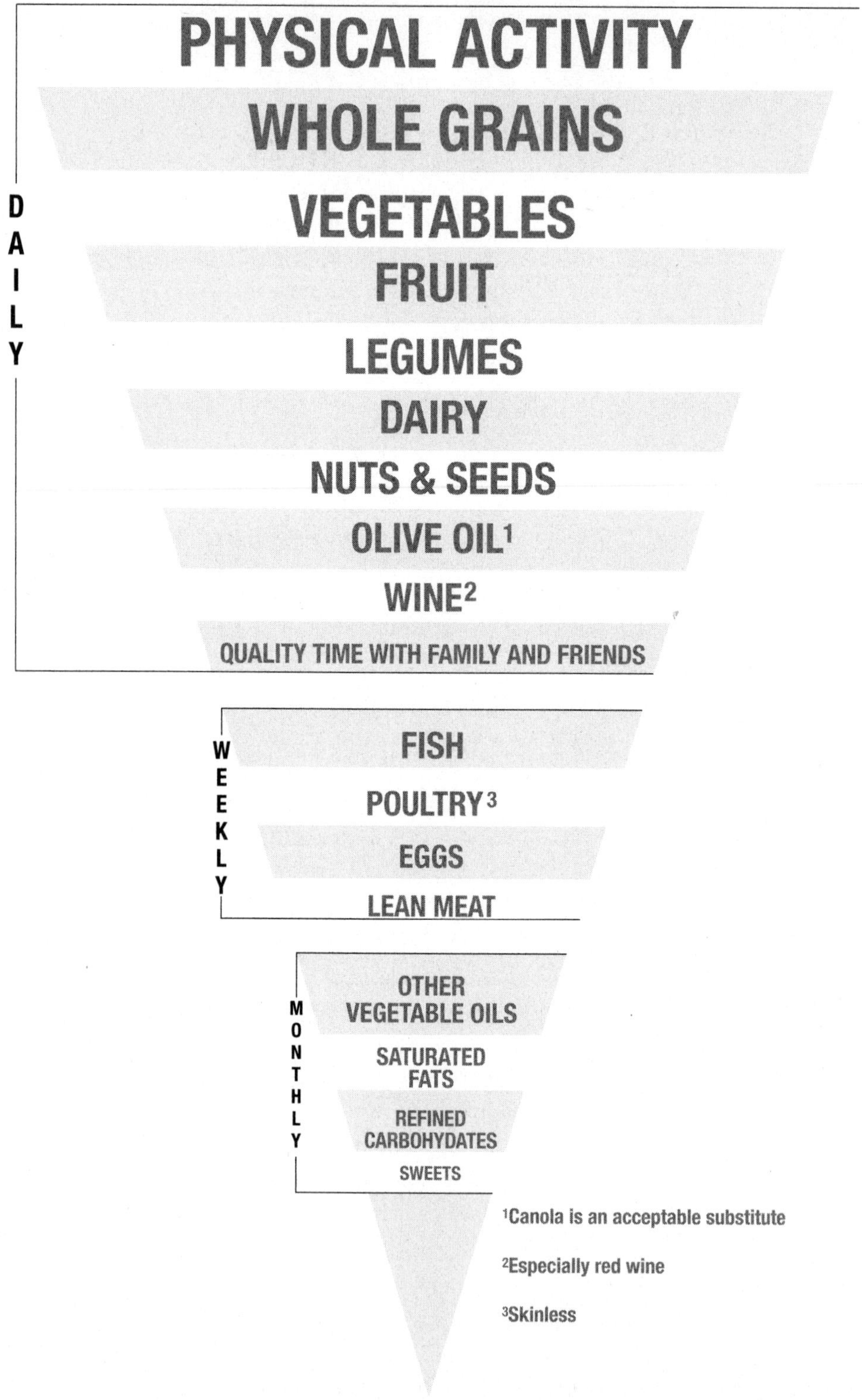

[1]Canola is an acceptable substitute

[2]Especially red wine

[3]Skinless

1. Eat Lots of Fruits

As a small child growing up in Sicily, I never had candy, cake, or ice cream for dessert. We fed our sweet tooths with natural treats—at the end of a meal, my mother would put out a large bowl of fruit and a bowl of nuts, and my father would crack the nuts, cut the fruit, and pass them around. Candy so easily brings a smile to children's faces that it's hard to deprive them of this simple joy. However, it would be vastly better to start them on the fresh fruit habit. Since what children eat is largely a matter of what's available, once they're used to fruit as a snack and dessert, they'll be just as happy with an orange as with the sugar and saturated fat of a candy bar. The same is true for grown-ups. To me, nothing could be a better dessert than a delicious ripe piece of in-season fruit, and I keep them well stocked at home and in my office. My habits have stayed with me since my childhood, and it's never too late to start.

A magnificent array of fruits grows in the Mediterranean region and are eaten as a sumptuous snack or sweet-tooth-satisfying dessert at the end of a meal. Fruits are full of essential vitamins and minerals, and most are high in vitamin C, a powerful antioxidant. Many also contain high amounts of carotenoids and other phytochemicals, health-promoting components that likely lend fruits their cancer-preventing qualities. Many studies have linked high fruit consumption (particularly in combination with high vegetable consumption, but also on their own) with lower cancer rates, especially of the digestive and respiratory tracts. While it may be that the protection against cancer weakens the farther from the digestive tract you get, significant protection is still seen for cancers of the liver, pancreas, prostate, breast, and urinary tract.

Fruits also help prevent cardiovascular disease—some studies suggest they may be even more effective than vegetables in this regard. In conjunction with high vegetable intake, fruits may also protect against diseases as varied as obesity, cataracts, diabetes, stroke, diverticulosis, Alzheimer's, and asthma. Deaths from all causes may be lower among those with daily fruit consumption, as suggested by a 2000 study that followed a group of about eight hundred men for over thirty years.

Fruits are also great sources of fiber, which not only helps you feel full but promotes long-term health. Fiber is the non-nutritive substance that gives plants their shape and sturdiness, but the body doesn't digest it as it goes through your system. **Fiber keeps your digestive and elimination systems running smoothly, and may keep your body from digesting some of the calories consumed as well.** High fiber intake has been linked to a decrease in certain cancers, may help diabetes patients by stabilizing blood sugar, and may lower LDL ("bad") cholesterol.

While you can't go wrong eating any fruit, they are not all created equal. Figure 1 shows antioxidant activity found in some common fruits.

Figure 1. Antioxidant Activity of Various Fruit Extracts

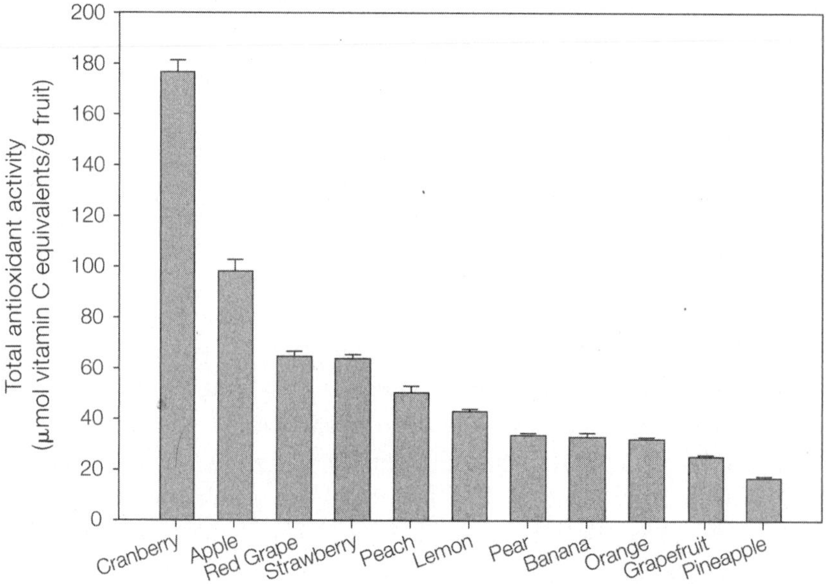

Reprinted from Jeanelle Boyer and Rui Hai Liu, "Apple Phytochemicals and Their Health Benefits," *Nutrition Journal* 2004, 3:5, available at http://www.nutritionj.com/content/3/1/5.

The old adage about eating an apple a day to keep the doctor away may well be true, as the humble apple is a powerhouse of phytochemicals and antioxidants. Their consumption alone has been linked with the reduction of some cancers (especially lung cancer), cardiovascular disease, asthma, and diabetes. In the laboratory, apples have been found to have strong antioxidant activity, inhibit cancer cell proliferation, decrease lipid oxidation, and lower cholesterol. Apple (as well as pear) intake has also been associated with weight loss. This may be due to the apple's rich supply of pectin, a type of soluble fiber that gels the cell walls of plants together. **In the digestive tract, ingested pectin helps slow down digestion, bestowing an appetite-suppressant effect and enabling you to feel full longer.** Take note, however, that the bulk of the apple's antioxidative power appears to reside in the peels, not so much in the flesh. This means that processed apple products, such as apple juice and applesauce, have nowhere near the anti-cancer and heart disease prevention effects that a whole apple would have. For example, apple juice may have as little as 3 percent of the antioxidant activity of a fresh apple. On the other hand, apple peels are so resilient, they can be blanched and freeze- or oven-dried and still maintain their strong antioxidant activity.

I recommend 3 to 4 servings of fruit per day, where one serving is equal to one piece of whole fruit, ½ cup of fresh or cooked fruit, 1 cup of high-water-content fruit such as melon or berries, or 2 to 4 tablespoons of dried fruit (raisins, apricots, dates, etc.). Fresh fruit is preferable, but there's nothing wrong with canned or frozen fruits, either, as long as there is no added sugar—try substituting frozen berries for ice cream. Try to eat a variety of different fruits. Choosing a different-colored fruit each time you select one helps ensure you are getting a variety of nutrients (see Appendix C). Personally, I prefer fruit, either fresh or dried, as a snack compared to vegetables; I feel like they're tastier and less boring, so I encourage you to indulge and get your phytochemicals there if you feel the same way. Eat a piece of fruit as a snack; even better, replace a dessert that's loaded with sugar and refined carbohydrates with something guilt-free and just as tasty, just as the Mediterraneans have done for centuries.

WAYS TO ADD MORE FRUIT INTO YOUR DAILY DIET

- Keep bowls of fresh fruit around at home; they're visually pleasing and will tempt you with the perfect snack.
- Bring fresh fruit to work so that a healthy snack is also the most convenient snack.
- Add a serving of fresh melon or citrus to your breakfast meal.
- Add a scrumptious pear, plum, peach, or apple to your lunch.

- Add some strawberries or grilled pears to your salad or have a beautiful bowl of mixed berries at dinner.
- Add raisins or other dried fruits to grain and meat dishes.
- Try different kinds of dried fruits as a snack—apricots, figs, dates, apples, blueberries, cranberries, and prunes are all delicious.

2. Eat Lots of Vegetables

Sicily was a poor region in Italy during the time I was growing up. Nevertheless, no matter how poor anyone was, everyone had at least a little plot of land. Everyone grew their own fruits and vegetables. So ingrained in them was this that my father insisted on buying his first house only five years after we moved to New York City from Sicily—and he wouldn't buy one unless it had a backyard in order to grow vegetables. As time went on, my father decided that the backyard wasn't big enough to grow his vegetables, so he bought a country house in upstate New York, where we still go to this day. There he has a one-acre garden lush with fruit trees, melons, cucumbers, beans, peppers, eggplants, tomatoes, and so on. In fact, all over America, Italian Americans are known for their beautiful backyard gardens and prize tomatoes! Everyone in our extended family helps maintain it, which is a labor of love for all of us. Spending time together working in the garden brings us together as a family. My philosophy is, if you spend time with the basketball hoop, you'll bond with the basketball hoop. I would rather bond with my family, doing things together and spending time together.

Modern Americans are not as ingrained with the vegetable habit, unfortunately, and they should be. You've heard it since you were a child, and I'm not going to tell you any differently: vegetables are really, really good for you. They are probably the most important element of the Mediterranean Prescription. Traditional Mediterranean cuisine abounds with vegetables—fresh, in-season, and in endless varieties. If you gradually replace some of your meat portion per meal, especially red meat, with more and more vegetables, you're already halfway toward staying slim permanently and improving your health immeasurably. You should consume **4 to 6 servings of vegetables (1 serving is about ½ cup cooked or 1 cup raw or leafy vegetables, or ¾ cup vegetable juice) every day.**

Nowhere are vitamins, minerals, phytochemicals, and antioxidants more densely concentrated than in vegetables. As with fruits, the concentration of antioxidants in vegetables prevents oxidative stress that contributes to many diseases. Numerous studies have established the protective effects of vegetables against certain chronic diseases, cancer (especially of the respiratory and digestive tracts, oral cavity, stomach, lung, pancreas, bladder, colon, cervix, ovary, and breast, as well as hormone-related tumors), stroke, and many functional declines associated with aging. For example, a 2004 study demonstrated that a diet that included 5 or more servings of a combination of fruit and vegetables per day lowered the risk of cardiovascular disease by 28 percent compared to diets with only 1½ servings. Furthermore, green leafy vegetables had the strongest specific association with decreased risk—with each additional serving per day, heart disease risk went down 11 percent more.

Besides fighting disease, vegetables can increase your life expectancy. In the many longitudinal studies that examined the association between vegetable intake and mortality, the striking finding is that virtually whatever the length of follow-up, whatever endpoint or age or sex considered, the results are incredibly similar: high vegetable intake can help extend your life. In a recent examination of 1,500 Italian men followed for thirty years, those who ate just a bare minimum amount of 60 grams per day of vegetables, as opposed to only 20 grams per day or less, lived two years longer. Interestingly, this protective effect was more pronounced for smokers than for nonsmokers (though smokers never attained the longevity that non-smokers did, regardless of vegetable consumption).

A QUICK PRIMER ON VEGETABLE TYPES

- **Cruciferous vegetables.** Cruciferous vegetables (so named because of the cross-shaped arrangement of their flower petals) are members of the cabbage family and should be a regular part of everyone's diet. Examples are broccoli, cauliflower, brussels sprouts, cabbage, arugula, bok choy, collard greens, kale, broccoli rabe, mustard greens, radishes, turnips, rutabaga, and watercress. These vegetables contain isothiocyanates, which stimulate our bodies to break down carcinogens, and antioxidants such as beta-carotene, vitamin C, and sulforaphane. Eating liberally from this vegetable group may help protect you from many cancers, including prostate, breast, ovarian, colorectal, and stomach. Broccoli alone—a virtual vegetable superstar—contains vitamins A and C, fiber, folate, calcium, iron, potassium, magnesium, beta-carotene, and a host of other phytochemicals. Cabbage also contains brassinin, which has been shown in animal studies to decrease tumors of the skin and breasts. Incidentally, cruciferous *sprouts*—such as the immature plants of broccoli and cauliflower—have been found to have ten to one hundred times the anti-cancer compounds of the mature plants that we usually eat, so it would be even better to add this form to your diet!

- **Solanaceous vegetables.** The plant family Solanaceae includes vegetables such as tomatoes, peppers, potatoes, and eggplant—all good sources of vitamins A and C and potassium. Tomatoes in particular are a great source of lycopene, an antioxidant phytochemical that reduces the risk of prostate cancer and some other cancers, as well as cardiovascular disease. Lycopene is more concentrated in tomato sauce and paste, which traditional Mediterranean and Italian cuisines are chock-full of. And because lycopene is fat-soluble, it becomes even more available to the body when tomatoes are cooked in a small amount of oil.

- **Umbelliferous vegetables.** This family of vegetables with umbrella-like leaves includes carrots, celery, fennel, parsnips, and the herbs parsley and cilantro. These vegetables are a rich source of vitamins A and C, beta-carotene, and many other phytonutrients, such as coumarins, monoterpenes, polyacetylenes, and psoralens—substances that provide benefits ranging from cancer protection to helping with skin disorders such as psoriasis. Scientists believe that to maximize their anticarcinogenic properties, it is best to combine different kinds of these vegetables.

- **Cucurbitaceous vegetables.** Cucurbitaceous vegetables are the vine-growing gourd and melon family. Examples include pumpkin, squash, cucumber, zucchini, watermelon, honeydew melon, and cantaloupe. They contain high levels of vitamins A and C, beta-carotene, phosphorous, fiber, and flavonoids.

- **Allium vegetables**. The allium family includes bulb vegetables such as onion, garlic, shallots, scallions, leeks, and chives. They contain a host of phytochemicals and may also have antibacterial properties in the body. As it turns out, in addition to garlic keeping vampires away, it may keep cancer away as well. Researchers at the National Cancer Institute recently reported that a diet with lots of vegetables from the allium group reduces the risk of prostate cancer by about half. Men in China have the lowest rate of prostate cancer in the world, and their diet rich in garlic, shallots, and onions may be one of the reasons. Allium consumption may also reduce the risk of breast, colon, gastric, and colorectal cancers. Additionally, it may promote cardiovascular health by helping lower blood lipids and blood pressure and acting as a natural anticlotting agent. Two points to keep in mind: (1) these vegetables lose some of their health benefits upon cooking, and (2) the disease-preventing compounds are primarily available in the plants themselves, not in supplement form.

In a paper published in 1992 that reviewed three hundred nutritional studies, it was found that fruit and vegetables provide significant protection from cancer. While there is certainly nothing wrong with canned and frozen vegetables, it appears that **raw, fresh vegetables offer the most consistent protection.** This is especially true for lettuce and other leafy greens, cruciferous vegetables, allium vegetables, tomatoes, and carrots, and to a lesser extent for potatoes as well.

THE GLYCEMIC INDEX: FACT AND FICTION

Potatoes have gotten a bad rap lately in the popular diet press due to a fixation on the much-talked-about glycemic index, and it's not quite fair. The glycemic index basically measures the extent to which a given food causes your blood sugar to rise. You could say it is a measure of how rapidly you digest starchy foods. The theory goes that by eating low-glycemic-index foods, you avoid blood sugar spikes from high-glycemic-index foods (which include high-starch foods such as refined carbohydrates and potatoes, or even vegetables with a lot of sugar, such as carrots) and also keep your hunger from getting out of control. What many people don't realize is that measuring glycemic load was created as a way to assess the sugar content of the diet for people with diabetes. It also assumes that everyone is insulin-resistant. Insulin is a powerful hormone that drives blood sugar into cells and also stimulates the liver to convert sugar into its storable form, glycogen. If someone becomes insulin-resistant, they aren't responding so readily to insulin in their bloodstream, so the body kicks out more and more insulin to maintain normal blood sugar levels. The resulting high insulin not only predisposes people to acquiring type 2 diabetes, as well as other health conditions, but may also stimulate the appetite and lower the amount of sugar that is burned off as energy, while increasing glycogen and fat stores.

The problem is, only a minority (around 25 percent) of the population is insulin-resistant and thus might benefit from watching the glycemic index values of his or her food. In addition, there is no set value for each food, since it is influenced by many factors: the degree to which it has been processed, preparation techniques such as chopping or grinding, how long it is cooked, the frequency of your meals, the amount of soluble fiber in your normal diet, and the other foods you are consuming at the same time. Essentially, the more processed and broken down a food is, such as from cooking, the faster it will be digested in your system. This is why whole grains are a lower-glycemic-index food, while white bread, white rice, and other refined carbohydrates (with the fiber stripped away) are high-glycemic-index. But you can see from the number of factors that affect glycemic load that choosing a single food based on the glycemic index is oversimplifying, because how fast you digest food depends on so many other things. In fact, in a study recently published in the *Journal of Human Nutrition and Metabolism*, it has been shown that when you compare a low-glycemic-index diet to a high-glycemic-index diet, the glycemic load turns out to be irrelevant, and the only factor that really matters to achieve weight loss is the same old diet basic you've heard about ever since you started worrying about how your jeans fit: calorie count.

WHAT MAKES FRUITS AND VEGETABLES SO HEALTHY

A diet rich in fruits and vegetables not only provides essential vitamins and minerals that your body does not produce on its own, but it provides hundreds of phytochemicals—possibly even twenty-five thousand or more. **Phytochemicals** are non-nutrient plant chemicals, such as carotenoids (for example, beta-carotene), flavonoids, isoflavonoids, and phenolic acids. Besides giving plants their different tastes and colors, they are health-enhancing.

They have been associated with the reduction of chronic disease, including reductions in high blood pressure, diabetes, Alzheimer's, heart disease, and especially cancer. Most of the health benefits related to phytochemicals have to do with their role as antioxidants in maintaining the health of body cells and tissues. It has been found that a complex combination of phytochemicals, attained through the consumption of a wide array of fruits and vegetables, is the best way to receive the health benefits. Supplemental vitamins and/or minerals cannot replace the benefits gained from a diet rich in fruits and vegetables.

In addition to increasing overall immunity, phytochemicals interfere with some processes that cause cancer. The development of cancer cells is a multistep process (involving oxidative damage, DNA damage, production of damaged cells, and so on), and antioxidant phytochemicals can help interrupt this process through such means as the regulation of gene expression in cell proliferation, cell differentiation of oncogenes and tumor suppressor genes, induction of cell-cycle arrest (apoptosis), stimulation of the immune system, and many others.

The role of antioxidants in the prevention of cardiovascular disease cannot be overstated; their actions are believed to be the primary mechanism by which fruits and vegetables in the diet yield their great protective effects upon the heart and vascular system. Their role in benefiting cholesterol levels is considered to be much more important than monitoring the amount of cholesterol you take in in your diet.

There are two types of lipoproteins that are particularly implicated in the development of heart disease, and you've probably heard a lot about them: **LDL** (low-density lipoprotein), the "bad" kind, and **HDL** (high-density lipoprotein), the "good" kind. LDL carries cholesterol around in the bloodstream to your tissues (think of the *L* as indicating that it *leaves* cholesterol in your body), whereas HDL binds to excess cholesterol in the cells and shuttles it out of the bloodstream and into the liver to be processed and eliminated (think of the *H* as indicating that it *hauls* that cholesterol away). One of the leading theories as to how LDL contributes to atherosclerosis, or hardening and clogging of the arteries, is that when this type of carrier's cholesterol is oxidized it becomes a target for free radicals (molecules with one unpaired electron). In this destabilized state it becomes "sticky" and is thus more easily deposited on the internal lining of blood vessels. Oxidized LDL is believed to cause damage to the walls of the arteries, which then allows plaque (consisting of fatty substances, cholesterol, cellular waste products, fibrin, and calcium) to accumulate, leading to hardening of the arteries. The plaque accumulation can occlude blood flow, leading to a heart attack or stroke. However, the good news is that dietary antioxidants, such as from fruits and vegetables, can get incorporated into LDL and become oxidized themselves (they give an electron to odxidized cholesterol), thus stabilizing the cholesterol.

Without sufficient antioxidant protection, free radical damage will accumulate over time, leading to chronic illnesses such as cancer, heart disease, arthritis, macular degeneration, and many diseases of aging. Just remember: numerous antioxidant studies have demonstrated that supplementation in the form of a pill is ineffective and sometimes even harmful. By far the best source for antioxidants is fresh fruits and vegetables.

NO ONE EVER GOT FAT EATING TOO MANY VEGETABLES

The beauty of most vegetables, in addition to their robust nutritional benefits, is, of course, their delightfully low calorie count (see Appendix D). While other diets recommend watching your glycemic load, filling up on low-calorie vegetables, irrespective of where they fall on the glycemic index, is a far more effective weight loss and weight maintenance strategy for the long term. It's simple: ***the more vegetables you eat, the less body fat you're likely to have.*** Nibble on fresh vegetables during the day when you're hungry, and if you get hungry again, eat some more. Not only does the big salad before your main meal make you too full to finish your entrée, but the fiber from your vegetables slows digestion down, so you'll feel full longer.

Again, concentrate on changing your proportions on the Mediterranean Prescription. Go slowly if you wish, over time replacing more and more of your meat portion with larger and larger salad, vegetable, legume, and grain portions. You'll have the taste and texture of the meats you crave, and you'll feel just as full and satisfied because you're eating the same volume of food—but with the added bonuses that you'll be healthier and lose weight. After a while this eating habit will become second nature and won't feel like a diet at all. Try the many delicious vegetable recipes in this book, and sample vegetables you've never tried before.

Some of my patients initially thought some of the vegetables included in my diet were "weird," until they tried the recipes and loved them. You'll never adopt the vegetable habit into your life if you don't eat and prepare vegetables you love—so be adventurous and make an effort to find them!

SOME TIPS ON ADDING MORE VEGETABLES INTO YOUR DAILY DIET

- **Mix vegetables into sauces and baked goods.** For example, add peas, asparagus, arugula, onions, chopped mushrooms, or even spinach into spaghetti sauce. Grated carrots or zucchini could be added to whole-grain breads, muffins, or pancakes.
- **Keep washed and precut fresh vegetables in your fridge or at work in easily accessible containers.** It may sound obvious, but I'm convinced that convenience is the key here—just buying bags of whole carrots and celery may well not go any further than growing your own mold colonies in the produce drawer. Prewashed baby carrots are a godsend: they may be a little more expensive, but if it will get you to snack nutritiously, it's worth it to spend the extra cents. You should be spending less money on meat on the Mediterranean Prescription anyway. Cherry or grape tomatoes are equally easy—just rinse and pop into your mouth. Keep tasty, healthy dips around as well, such as eggplant dip or hummus. You could also drizzle olive oil over fresh vegetables and add a sprinkling of grated cheese or red pepper flakes if you wish. Remember to count your snacks as part of your daily servings.
- **Add a salad before your lunch or dinner, or as a snack.** Note that it's better to eat your salad before the entrée, the Mediterranean way, rather than with it, since you will fill up on the healthiest components of your meal. Your body needs a little time to register that your stomach is full, so starting out low-cal will prevent you from eating

more calories when you get to your entrée. Prewashed and prepackaged greens greatly reduce the barrier to fixing yourself a salad, so I highly recommend them. Once again, if it helps you get to a healthier, happier, thinner self, how could a few dollars here or there be better spent? Another option is to start your lunch or dinner with a colorful spread of crudités: spring onions, grape tomatoes, broccoli and cauliflower pieces, and carrots lightly drizzled with an olive oil vinaigrette.

- **Eat a vegetable-based soup before your lunch or dinner, or as a snack.** Once again, the high-volume, low-calorie formula is a great way to feel full and maintain a healthy weight. Bear in mind, though, that cream-based soups, even with vegetables such as broccoli, can be very high in caloric content. Try some of the tasty soup recipes in this book. For convenience, make a large portion, then freeze it in individual plastic containers, and microwave it as you go.
- **Experiment with different ways of cooking vegetables and with different recipes.** Your aversion to some vegetables may be conquered with just a revision in preparation. For example, try steaming vegetables instead of boiling: not only do you avoid the soggy-vegetable syndrome, you maintain a good deal more of their nutrients.
- **Simply prepare more vegetables than you usually do, and serve yourself a bigger portion.** If you tend to eat whatever's on your plate, manage what you put there instead of trying to manage your appetite. You may surprise yourself at how full and satisfied you can feel with a heaping portion of that "diet food."
- **Eat vegetables that are in season and fresh,** like the Mediterraneans do. As I've noted, the evidence suggests that fresh vegetables are the best for you—and they'll taste the best, too.

- **Make vegetable-based entrées a few times a week.** Try stuffed peppers or cabbage, a bean-and-vegetable-based stew, or pasta with a red sauce full of colorful vegetables.
- **Make an entrée of a large salad.** Add fish or beans if you like.
- **Frozen vegetables** are a great substitute when you are pressed for time. You can add them to sauces or just pop them in the microwave to cook. The beauty of frozen vegetables is that they are always around, even when the fresh version isn't in season. Just think of corn on the cob in the middle of the winter or winter squash in the early spring. My advice is still to make an effort to use fresh vegetables because you'll enjoy the flavor more, but many frozen vegetables are an acceptable alternative.
- **Canned vegetables** come in handy and save money. Adding mixed canned vegetables to your soups cuts down on the cooking time, and canned tomato products are essential in making many Mediterranean-style sauces. If the convenience of these items helps you to increase your vegetable intake, go for it. However, again, you may be less likely to tire of eating vegetables when you're using fresh ones, since they taste so good!

3. *Eat Lots of Legumes (Such as Beans, Peas, and Lentils)*

When I was growing up in Sicily, we would have some kind of legume every day—mostly lentils, chickpeas, pinto beans, or fava beans. We grew them in our garden, as did all of our neighbors. We lived in a congenial environment where when one person's garden didn't yield all of the crops they desired, a neighbor would likely offer what was missing. For instance, for some reason we never grew fava beans very well, but my father loved them, so people were always bringing us fava beans. This wonderful, neighborly arrangement meant that we always had a wide variety of vegetables and legumes, which we know now is a key to good health. My family and I still grow several legumes at our country home today.

Legumes are consumed quite frequently in the Mediterranean and are an important component of the Mediterranean Prescription. They are, technically, any of a large number of plant species with seed pods that split along both sides when ripe. Some of the more common ones are beans (any kind, such as string, yellow, fava, lima, and pinto), peas, lentils (yellow, red, and green), peanuts, garbanzo beans (chickpeas), and soybeans. Legumes are rich sources of fiber, B vitamins, folic acid, minerals, antioxidants, complex carbohydrates, and protein. They are also inexpensive and easy to incorporate into your favorite dishes, as you can easily mix them into soups, salads, and main courses. We recommend **2 or more ½-cup servings a day;** if this seems like too much for your taste, try for a minimum of a ½-cup or larger portion five or more times a week.

Many people don't want to bother with the process of cooking legumes. While they are relatively easy to cook, most do take some soaking and boiling time. Canned beans are a great time-saver here. They are already cooked and can be added to salads, pasta dishes, and made into wonderful entrées straight from the can. Lentils, which aren't generally canned, are very easy to cook—they boil up in about twenty to thirty minutes.

Legumes can be used in place of meat—and often are in Mediterranean cuisine. In fact, ½ cup of cooked dried beans has the same amount of protein as 1 ounce of meat, but none of the saturated fat. Calorie-wise, our serving recommendations are based on the idea that you would be replacing some of your normal meat consumption with legumes (the calorie count for ½ cup of beans is equivalent to 3 ounces of lean meat). Apart from the health benefit of reducing red meat in your diet, legumes will also help lower your cholesterol and lessen your risk of cardiovascular and heart disease, as well as your risk of osteoporosis. They also have a low glycemic index, so they're of benefit to those with insulin resistance or diabetes.

Some researchers believe that legumes are actually the most important component of a healthy Mediterranean diet and account for the longer life people on the diet have. A recent study of almost eight hundred people age seventy and older showed that across cultures (Japan, Sweden, Australia, and Greece), for every 20 grams of legumes you consume daily, you reduce your risk of death by around 8 percent over seven years. Despite the different varieties of legumes the cultures consume, the life span benefits were present: Japanese eat soy, tofu, natto, and miso; Swedes eat a lot of brown beans and peas; the Mediterranean people eat lentils, chickpeas, and white beans. Furthermore, in a significant number of the studies cited in the 1992 review I mentioned earlier, legume consumption was also found to offer protection from cancer.

THE HOMOCYSTEINE FACTOR

Medical researchers have linked a substance in the blood called homocysteine to a higher risk of heart disease. Homocysteine is an amino acid that naturally occurs in the body and is a by-product of protein intake, mostly from meat. It gets broken down by folic acid (also called folate and folacin), vitamin B_6, and vitamin B_{12}. When homocysteine fails to get broken down properly, it accumulates to high levels in the blood. In recent years, **elevated blood levels of homocysteine have been strongly associated with increased risk of premature coronary artery disease, stroke, and thromboembolism (blood clots in the veins),** even among people who have normal cholesterol levels. Reports suggest that some 10 to 30 percent of cases of heart disease are linked to elevated homocysteine levels. Indeed, it's likely that homocysteine plays some role in any disease where arteries are important, such as some kinds of dementia. Despite all of the copious data supporting the connection, scientists still do not understand the role of homocysteine completely, and many studies are currently under way to try to explain the mechanism. It's believed that when homocysteine levels rise, the walls of the arteries become "sticky," catching blood cholesterol and encouraging the accumulation of plaque. This accumulation can eventually result in hardening of the arteries and/or artery blockage. If you're concerned about your own level, it can be measured by a simple blood test at your doctor's office.

While no studies have proven that lowering homocysteine levels ultimately helps reduce strokes, heart attacks, and other cardiovascular events, it is a good idea to lower a high homocysteine level because of its substantial association with heart disease. Because **folic acid and vitamins B_6 and B_{12} break down homocysteine,** you should be sure to get enough in your diet, especially if you're at risk of a coronary event. If adjusting your diet is not enough to lower your homocysteine, your physician may recommend that you take folic acid and a vitamin B_6 supplement, which many cardiologists now do. For the general population, however, the American Heart Association, like the Mediterranean Prescription, doesn't recommend widespread use of supplements such as folic acid and B vitamins to reduce the risk of heart disease and stroke; rather, they advise a healthy, balanced diet that includes at least five servings of fruits and vegetables a day. Legumes such as lentils, chickpeas, and most beans are great sources of folic acid and vitamin B_6, as are dark green leafy vegetables such as kale, spinach, and some lettuces.

LEGUMES AND WEIGHT LOSS

In addition to the great health benefits of legumes in the diet, the abundant fiber and protein present in these foods go a long way toward helping you feel full following a meal and beyond. A 2005 report in *Nutrition* noted, "The average fiber intake of adults in the United States is less than half the recommended levels and is lower still among those who follow currently popular low-carbohydrate diets, such as Atkins and South Beach. Increasing consumption of dietary fiber with fruits, vegetables, whole grains, and legumes across the life cycle is a critical step in stemming the epidemic of obesity found in developed countries. The addition of functional fiber to weight-loss diets should be considered as a tool to improve success." Basically, **fiber intake is inversely associated with body weight and body fat.** Many mechanisms have been suggested for how dietary fiber aids in weight management, including helping you feel full, preventing your digestive system from absorbing all the calories you eat by adding bulk and speeding up transit time, and altering secretion of gut hormones.

Protein is as hunger-conquering as fiber. Studies suggest that **protein is more satiating than carbohydrate and fat,** and legumes are protein-rich. An illustration of its weight-loss benefits comes from a study in which participants who went on a diet high in soy protein and low in fat for six months lost a significant amount of weight. The study also demonstrated that this diet could improve body composition in overweight and obese people, who lost fat but preserved muscle mass. As you will read in the physical activity section below, preserving muscle mass during weight loss is key, since muscle burns calories at such a high rate.

Note, however, that you can't eat legumes with the abandon you can vegetables, because legumes are higher in calories. For example, ½ cup chickpeas is 135 calories, ½ cup lentils is 115, and ½ cup navy beans is 228; compare this to ½ cup broccoli at 22 calories and ½ cup zucchini slices at 14. So it's more important to stick to our serving size suggestions. Additionally, while most legumes are only about 1 percent fat by weight, soybeans are 18 to 20 percent fat (composed of 15 percent saturated, 23 percent monounsaturated, and 58 percent polyunsaturated; you'll read more about these fats a little further on). This means you have to watch the amount of soybeans more than other legumes.

SOME TIPS FOR ADDING MORE LEGUMES TO YOUR DAILY DIET

- Mix beans or lentils into meat dishes, sauces, and casseroles.
- Gradually increase the proportion of beans and lentils while decreasing the amount of meat ingredients.
- Add kidney or pinto beans to taco fillings and burritos.
- Try canned chickpeas over salads.
- Stir frozen peas into a casserole.
- Add twice the amount of kidney beans to chili (and, even better, use no or less red meat).
- Add black-eyed peas to homemade or canned soup.
- Try hummus as a dip with fresh vegetables or whole-wheat pita bread the next time you want a snack.
- Have a bean dip with fresh vegetables, whole-wheat pita bread, or crackers made with stone-ground whole grains as an appetizer.

- Snack on roasted beans, such as soy nuts.
- Try my Lentil Soup, one of my patients' favorite recipes; it makes a large quantity, so you can refrigerate or freeze the extra and keep it on hand.
- Prepare Mediterranean-style pasta and beans for an entrée.

4. Eat Lots of Nuts and Seeds

We were fortunate in Sicily that because of the hot climate and the type of land, we could always have fresh nuts such as almonds and walnuts. While California is a large producer of almonds in the United States, it's a lot less common in this country to have such access to fresh nuts. We would go to the country and shake the trees for the almonds and walnuts to drop down—the black skins of the walnuts would stain everyone's hands. We would then have our stockpile of nuts for the rest of the winter and the next season. As I mentioned earlier, I fondly remember my father cracking the nuts open after a meal for all the kids and passing them around. He still does that to this day for his grandchildren.

Nuts and seeds are a rich source of many vitamins, minerals, phytochemicals, antioxidants, and of plant protein, and no healthy diet should be without them. Epidemiologic research (studies of populations over time) consistently shows that frequent consumption of nuts (5 or more ounces per week) is associated with a 30 to 50 percent decrease in coronary heart disease. Researchers believe this is because of the unsaturated fat and fiber content working together to improve blood cholesterol and triglyceride levels, decrease platelet aggregation, and prevent heart arrhythmias. The minerals in nuts, such as magnesium and potassium, may help to lower high blood pressure as well. All of these benefits are also important for type 2 diabetics and those with insulin resistance who are at risk of developing diabetes. In point of fact, a large 2002 study that was reported in the *Journal of the American Medical Association* demonstrated that higher consumption of nuts, and even peanut butter, was associated with a lower risk of type 2 diabetes, irrespective of other risk factors. In separate studies, higher intakes of magnesium, fiber, and foods with a low glycemic index (which nuts have) all contribute to a reduced risk of type 2 diabetes, so this is no doubt related to the protective mechanism involved.

Some of the many benefits of nuts:

- Studies consistently show that frequent nut consumption may be protective against coronary heart disease and heart attack.
- Nuts are a rich source of protein and fiber, both of which help you feel full for long periods of time.
- Nuts have high amounts of the health-promoting substances magnesium, vitamin E, potassium, calcium, zinc, selenium, and arginine.
- Most nuts have "good fats"—monounsaturated fats and polyunsaturated fats, including (especially in walnuts) alpha-linolenic acid, which is an omega-3 fatty acid found in vegetable sources.
- Nuts and seeds may help protect women from colorectal cancer.
- No preparation is necessary; you can keep them at the office or in the car as a handy, healthy snack.

While nuts are 70 to 80 percent fat, most of the fat is unsaturated fat (poly- and monounsaturated), which is the "good" kind. Coconut, however, is very high in saturated fat and should be avoided. For the rest, calorie counts should be somewhat kept in mind, since nuts and seeds are relatively high in calories (see the table on page 38). Thus I recommend a smaller daily quantity than other components in the Mediterranean Prescription: **1 ounce of nuts and seeds per day** (the equivalent of about twenty-four almonds), eaten plain or as an addition to other food items. Hopefully you'll be trimming calories in other areas on the Mediterranean Prescription—by reducing your intake of meat, as well as higher-fat dairy and other foods high in saturated fat—so eating nuts and seeds will not be adding extra calories to your daily diet.

Calorie counts do not appear to be strictly relevant with nuts, though, since **several studies have shown that nuts added to a diet do not cause weight gain. Some subjects even lose weight when they add nuts to their diet.** A recent study with walnuts supported these results, where calorie intake rose when walnuts were added, but no weight gain was seen.

In another study, researchers at Purdue University found that adding almonds to a calorie-controlled eating plan assisted in weight loss. Although the study was short-term and small in sample size, it does demonstrate that people were able to eat nuts and lose weight. It's not known exactly why nuts have this effect, though it's possible that the satiation nuts provide from their fiber, protein, and fat prevents overeating at other times, or that certain types of fatty acids are processed differently when they are consumed in foods as opposed to in oils.

Sunflower, pumpkin, and sesame seeds can be added to your diet as a tasty snack or as a crunchy addition to salads, side dishes, or entrées. Sunflower seeds are packed with nutrients including vitamin E, thiamine, magnesium, and vitamin B_6. Eat sunflower seeds with foods rich in beta-carotene and vitamin C, like fruits and tomatoes, to aid in iron absorption. Pumpkin seeds may help protect you from heart disease and high blood pressure due to their alpha-linolenic acid content. Like nuts, their fat content is high, but mostly unsaturated. This may help in lowering high serum cholesterol. Again, eating the seeds with foods high in beta-carotene and vitamin C will aid in iron absorption. They can be consumed with or without the shell. Sesame is another type of seed in which most of the fat is unsaturated. These flavorsome seeds contain magnesium for steadying nerves (great for any dieter) and zinc to strengthen immunity, plus they do wonders in perking up the flavors of other foods.

NUTS AND SEEDS

Nut or Seed (Dried or dry-roasted)	Serving Size	Total Fat (g)	Saturated Fat (g)	Calories
Almonds	1 oz (24)	15	1	165
Cashews	1 oz (18)	13	2.6	165
Chestnut, European	1 oz (3½)	0.6	0.1	70
Hazelnuts	1 oz (¼ cup)	17.3	1.3	175
Macadamia nuts	1 oz (11)	21	3	200
Mixed nuts	1 oz	14.6	2	170

Nut or Seed (Dried or dry-roasted)	Serving Size	Total Fat (g)	Saturated Fat (g)	Calories
Peanut butter	1 oz (2 Tbsp.)	14.2	2.7	170
Peanuts	1 oz (36)	14	2	160
Pecans	1 oz (31)	19	1.5	190
Pine nuts	1 oz	17.3	2.6	180
Pistachios	1 oz (47)	14	1.5	165
Pumpkin seeds	⅓ cup	5	1	110
Sesame seeds, whole	1 oz	13.5	2	160
Sunflower seeds or kernels	1 oz	14	1.5	160
Walnuts	1 oz (¼ cup)	18.3	1.1	200

Personally, I like to have a small handful of nuts as a hunger quencher in between meals. For example, if I'm going out to dinner, I'll often have about eight almonds before I go so that I'm not too hungry when I get to dinner and won't subsequently overeat. I also keep nuts at the office to stave off hunger. I might eat ten to fourteen nuts, especially before I go to the gym. I usually get a bit hungry around four o'clock every afternoon. If I have a craving for something unhealthy, I'll have a small handful of nuts and the craving goes away, and I forget that I was hungry for whatever it was.

WAYS TO ADD NUTS AND SEEDS INTO YOUR DAILY DIET

- Sprinkle almonds on your salad at any meal.
- Walnuts are a crunchy, nutty addition to pasta dishes.

- Have a handful of mixed nuts or seeds as a filling and delicious snack.
- Pesto with pine nuts on pasta is a delicious Mediterranean meal.
- Have some nut butter on bread for dessert. Peanut butter is good (made with unsaturated fat), but you must try almond butter, walnut butter, or cashew butter for a tasty delight.

5. Eat a Lot of Whole Grains, Especially Whole-Grain Bread

When I was growing up in Sicily, we never bought bread in the store. My mother always made it. I'd get home from school about three o'clock and she'd always slice a piece of bread hot out of the oven for me. She'd pour olive oil on the bread, and that was my snack. The bread was the most wonderful consistency—it was dark brown with a dense, grainy texture, not like the fluffy bread in the United States. A slice really filled you up. If you picked up a loaf of my mother's bread, you could get a hernia, it's that dense. Little did she know at the time how healthy it was for her family. To preserve this tradition, I actually built a brick oven in our country house and in my apartment in New York City.

Whole grains are emphasized in both the Mediterranean diet and the diet suggested by the modern USDA Food Guide Pyramid. They are generally low in saturated fat and have a high content of nutrients that are related to beneficial health effects, such as fiber, vitamins (especially vitamin E and B vitamins), minerals (calcium, magnesium, potassium, phosphorous, selenium, manganese, zinc, and iron), antioxidants, phytoestrogens, and a wide range of other phytochemicals that have been associated with long-term health. They are considered so important to health that in both pyramids—in fact, in most dietary pyramids out there—they take the most prominent position on the triangle: the first level, the constituent of the diet that should be consumed the most. **I recommend eating a full 8 servings of whole grains each day** for maximal health. This can be in the form of whole-grain breads, pasta, cereal, rice, bulgur, couscous, polenta, and many others. One serving is equal to one ounce of dry grain (which equals one slice of bread, 1/2 cup cooked grains or pasta, or 3/4 cup dry or 1/2 cup cooked cereal).

THE WHOLE-GRAIN ADVANTAGE

A distinction must be made between whole-grain and refined-grain foods. A whole grain consists of three botanically defined parts: the **bran**, the **germ**, and the **endosperm**. The bran and germ contain many nutrients and phytochemicals and a lot of fiber, whereas the endosperm is largely starch and provides mostly energy (calories). Milling strips off most of the bran and germ and pulverizes the endosperm. The resulting refined grains are digested more quickly than whole-grain products and thus tend to cause more rapid and larger increases in blood glucose and insulin.

SOME COMMON GRAINS

Maximize	Minimize
Whole-wheat bread	White bread
Brown rice	White rice
Whole-wheat and semolina-based pastas	Refined-flour pastas
Whole-wheat flour	White flour
Multigrain breads	White bread, white dinner rolls, white-flour bagels, most cookies, cakes, and doughnuts
Whole oats (steel-cut oats, rolled oats, old-fashioned oats)	Instant oatmeal and other quick cooking oats
Bran muffin	Smooth-textured breakfast muffins
Rice cakes made from brown rice	Rice cakes made from white rice
Whole-grain cornmeal/polenta	Corn flour
Barley	

Intake of whole grains, especially whole-grain bread, is associated with a broad array of health benefits. Studies suggest a 20 to 30 percent decrease in coronary heart disease occurs with a daily intake of three or more servings of whole-grain foods, likely due to the fiber content, as well as the antioxidant activity of the phytochemicals in whole grains (probably especially in the bran, though this is not yet known for certain). Type 2 diabetes is also less frequent among people who eat a diet rich in whole grains. Insulin resistance, the asymptomatic precursor to diabetes, is ameliorated by whole-grain foods as well. Even when you look at mortality from all causes, whole-grain eaters are shown to do better. One study showed that all-cause mortality was 23 percent lower in the group that ate the most whole grains when compared to the group that ate the least.

In contrast, refined grains are typically calorie-rich and nutrient-poor. High consumption of refined grains is also associated with increased risk of atherosclerosis, coronary artery disease, and all-cause mortality.

The consumption of whole grains in America is abysmally low, as it is in many industrialized nations. In most developed countries, cereal grains are generally highly processed before use. In 1997 in the United States, only 2 percent of the 150 pounds of wheat flour consumed per person was whole-wheat; the rest was refined. Consumption of less-refined grains has no doubt increased since then with increased publicity about the healthfulness of whole grains, but even in 2003 the average consumption of whole-grain foods was 1 serving per day; a mere 8 percent of U.S. adults consume 3 servings per day. This is just fine with the food companies. In the same way food manufacturers turn healthy fats into trans fats to increase the shelf life of their goods, food companies process grains so they'll last longer, too. During milling the germ is usually separated from the rest of the wheat grain because its fat content limits the shelf life of the flour. But the germ is the part of the grain that would sprout if it was planted as a seed, and it's packed with nutrients and protein with which to nourish a new plant. Luckily, food companies are getting the message that people want more of these wholesome foods. Watch the market for a whole new array of whole-grain products.

FIBER

Fiber is the indigestible and non-nutritive part of plants. There are two types: insoluble and soluble. **Insoluble fiber** does not dissolve in water, so it helps the body to regulate bowel function by adding bulk. **Soluble fiber** partially dissolves in water and forms a sticky gel that may sweep harmful substances from the intestines. While, contrary to past thinking, recent large studies have shown little evidence that fiber protects against colon cancer, we do know that fiber provides many other health benefits. There is evidence that fiber helps to reduce cholesterol levels and that it may decrease the risk of developing heart disease, diabetes, diverticular disease, irritable bowel syndrome, certain other cancers, and constipation.

Adding fiber to your diet can help you lose weight. As I've noted before, fiber makes you feel full both during a meal, so you stop eating sooner, and after a meal, so you can go longer without becoming hungry again. (This is somewhat moreso for soluble fiber than for insoluble fiber.) Some studies show that people eat a constant weight of food rather than a constant number of calories. With this in mind, replacing high-fat foods with high-fiber foods would be a good weight-loss strategy. You'll consume fewer calories and feel just as full and satisfied. Even the textural quality of fiber may help, since it slows down chewing, prolonging eating time and thus giving the feeling of fullness a chance to kick in. Research also shows that soluble fiber in particular may reduce the number of calories absorbed by getting in the way of fat (and possibly carbohydrate) absorption.

SOURCES OF FIBER

Soluble Fiber	Insoluble Fiber
Oatmeal	Whole grains such as whole-wheat breads, couscous, brown rice, and bulgur
Oat bran	Wheat bran
Nuts and seeds	Whole-grain breakfast cereals
Legumes such as dried peas, beans, and lentils	Vegetables such as carrots, cucumbers, zucchini, celery, and tomatoes
Fruits such as apples, pears strawberries, and blueberries	Seeds
Vegetables such as eggplant and okra	
Barley	

I recommend that adults eat 20 to 35 grams of fiber a day, which should include both soluble and insoluble fiber. (For children over age two, the recommended intake is the child's age plus 5 grams.) Achieving this amount of fiber is doable if you are following the Mediterranean Prescription. Some examples of fiber content: 1 apple has 4 grams, 3 dried figs have 11 grams, ½ cup broccoli provides 4 grams, ½ cup chickpeas has 6 grams, ½ cup kidney beans has 10 grams, 1 slice of whole-grain bread has 3 grams, 1 cup cooked whole-wheat spaghetti contains 6 grams, and ½ cup brown rice provides 6 grams.

GRAINS AND WEIGHT LOSS

Whole-grain and fiber-rich diets have been associated with weight loss and a lower risk of obesity. Essentially, the high fiber content of most whole-grain foods may help prevent weight gain by increasing appetite control and by preventing the complete calorie absorption of a meal.

A few fairly large recent studies have shown that as whole-grain intake goes up, weight gain goes down. In studies at the University of Minnesota, slight reductions in weight were observed in subjects fed identical-calorie diets with the only difference being whole grains versus refined grains. While the weight loss was not statistically significant after only six weeks, it suggests that long-term consumption may support weight reduction. The bran in whole-grain foods may be a key (but not the only) component, as adding bran to the diet has been shown to further reduce the risk of weight gain. In contrast, weight gain goes up as intake of refined-grain foods increases.

One thing to keep in mind when you are trying to lose weight is that **whole grains can contribute significantly to total calorie intake.** Thus the recommended serving sizes should not be exceeded, and the grains should be consumed as specified if you are on my weight loss plan. Whole grains are carbohydrates, albeit complex ones. Since most people get about 60 percent of their total calories from carbohydrates, it makes sense that to lose weight you need to watch this component of your diet. It is interesting to note that over the past several decades, as America was getting fatter, carbohydrates became a larger portion of our diet, while fat and protein consumption decreased.

CARBOHYDRATES

Carbohydrates are composed of chains of sugar units and come in two basic forms: simple and complex. Simple carbs are one, two, or at most three units of sugar linked together in single molecules, while in complex carbs hundreds or thousands of sugar units can be linked together in single molecules. Simple carbs are easily identified by their taste, which is sweet. Complex carbs, such as potatoes, are pleasant to the taste but are not sweet. After digestion, both types of carbohydrates appear in the circulatory system as the sugar glucose, where it proceeds to the cells and is used for energy.

There are three main types of carbohydrates:

1. **Sugars**
2. **Starches**
3. **Fiber**

SUGAR

Carbohydrates that contain only one sugar unit (monosaccharides) or two sugar units (disaccharides) are referred to as simple sugars (or simple carbohydrates). Simple sugars are broken down quickly in the body to release energy. Two of the most common monosaccharides are glucose and fructose: glucose is the primary form of sugar stored in the human body for energy, whereas fructose is the main sugar found in most fruits. A common disaccharide is sucrose, which is what table sugar is.

STARCH

Starch is a complex carbohydrate made from thousands of glucose molecules linked together (polysaccharide). Starch is the main compound that plants use to store their food energy and is found in the innermost part (endosperm) of the seed or grain. Starch is found in plant-based foods, especially cereals, bread, potatoes, corn, legumes (beans), pasta, and rice. Starch is also found in some fruits and vegetables.

FIBER

Fiber, or cellulose, is another important polysaccharide. Cellulose is a structural molecule that adds support to plant leaves, stems, and other parts. Because of its stronger structure and stability compared to sugars and starches, cellulose cannot be digested by human beings. See more on fiber in the box above.

WAYS TO ADD WHOLE GRAINS TO YOUR DAILY DIET

- Have a slice of crunchy whole-grain Italian bread or chewy whole-wheat pita bread for breakfast. You can spread it with a nut butter like almond butter or top it with some fresh sliced peaches for sweetness.
- Have whole-grain porridge as an old-world breakfast. Oats, rolled wheat, stone-ground cornmeal, or barley cereals are whole-grain favorites to try.
- Make an herbed brown-rice risotto or pilaf to serve with your lunch entrée.
- Pasta, in its amazing variety, is a wonderful addition to dinner. The different shapes and varieties of pasta all have their own unique texture and flavor. Many varieties are available in a whole-wheat version. Serve your pasta with a vegetable-and-olive-oil-based sauce (not cream-based, which is very high in calories).
- Polenta made with stone-ground cornmeal is a favorite with any meal.
- Add a slice of herbed whole-grain focaccia or crusty ciabatta to your meal.
- Cook brown rice as a pilaf or risotto, or add it to soup.

6. *Use Olive Oil Liberally, Both in Salads and in Cooking*

I never knew what butter was until I moved to America. Everyone used olive oil in Sicily, and everyone made their own. We would put sheets on the ground under the trees and shake the olives off the trees. Then we'd gather up the sheets with the olives and bring the fruit to the local mill, which would process them for us. That was the source of the olive oil we used throughout the year.

The oil was very, very dark green, with a thick consistency; you could hardly see through the bottle. It was so dense with flavor and fragrance that you could smell the aroma as it was coming out of the bottle. The taste was equally strong. Unlike the milder olive oils you usually get in the United States, this oil kept its flavor when you cooked it. In fact, I so much prefer the rich flavor and quality of this oil that to this day my relatives still send my family oil in ten-gallon drums from Sicily.

It's funny, but Sicilians think olive oil and garlic will cure everything. They use the oil as a laxative, for headaches or indigestion, as a skin moisturizer, and so forth. In addition, they think all ailments are caused by eating. When someone died, I'd ask my mother, "What did he die from?" "I don't know," she'd say. "One day he ate a bowl of lentils, and he dropped dead." They always attribute it to what they had for lunch or dinner that day.

Olive cultivation dates back to biblical times. The farming of the olive tree and the production of olive oil from the mature fruit remain an essential part of agricultural practices in the Mediterranean basin today. Olive oil is a vital component of the Mediterranean Prescription, and some even argue that it's the most important factor in the disease-fighting, life-prolonging effects of following a traditional Mediterranean diet. When Ancel Keys, the distinguished researcher, was comparing diets in different parts of the globe, he found Mediterranean cuisine to be the healthiest, and the Greek island of Crete, in particular, to have the lowest rates of heart disease and many other chronic disorders. The Cretans also had the highest consumption of olive oil in the study: about ½ cup a day per person! This was a full one-third of their daily calories. Interestingly, they were also the leanest group of the seven countries studied. I don't recommend quite that much olive oil, however, since most people in the United States aren't toiling in the fields all day and burning all that off like the Cretans were. You should **use olive oil daily,** around 2 to 4 tablespoons depending on your caloric needs, both in salads and in cooking. There are other healthy oils out there (see the fats section), but personally, olive oil is all I cook with, bake with, scramble eggs with, and use for salad dressings. You can even drizzle it on bread or dip your bread into it, and do away with butter and margarine altogether.

Besides the decadently rich taste of olive oil, you should also be using it, of course, for your health. Olive oil has been shown to help protect against heart disease, heart attack, cancer (colon, breast, and skin), and aging. It also may help lower high blood pressure, benefit blood cholesterol levels (raise the good kind and lower the bad), improve diabetes, and boost your immune response. The therapeutic properties of olive oil have been attributed to its **high level of monounsaturated fat,** though this does not appear to be the whole story. Some speculate the many protective effects of olive oil are due to its powerful, free-radical-scavenging antioxidants such as phenolic compounds, vitamin E, and carotenoids. Oleic acid, a monounsaturated fat and also a powerful antioxidant, is the main component of olive oil and may be responsible for suppressing oncogenes (genes having the potential to cause normal cells to become cancerous).

Olive oil can be a healthy source of fat in a weight loss plan. A recent study examined men on a diet with 40 percent of calories from fat—the typical American diet—in which one group had a high saturated-fat intake and the other consumed more monounsaturated fats. Eating the same amount of calories, the monounsaturated-fat dieters lost weight while the other group didn't. It is speculated that this may happen because saturated fat has a higher propensity to be stored as body fat rather than be burned for energy, as monounsaturated fat is.

Studies show people don't stick to low-fat diets, and they don't have to. Aim for 30 to 35 percent of your total calories from fat (only 10 percent or less of that should come from saturated fats). This is what works in the long term, as a lifestyle, to keep you healthy and lean. Most people can't stick to no carbs or low carbs for their lives, either, and again, they don't have to. Fat gives flavor and texture to food, and we're programmed to enjoy that. By eating healthy fats and giving up unhealthy ones, you win twice: you're healthier and thinner. Just remember that when introducing olive oil into your diet, you have to compensate by removing other fats, particularly any animal sources of fat, such as butter or fat from red meat.

The first thing to reduce in your diet is the use of table spreads like butter and margarine. If you must use them, trans-fat-free canola-oil-based soft margarines are an acceptable option on the Mediterranean diet. However, instead of using those on your breads, you may wish to dip your bread in olive oil. In cooking, olive oil is the best fat for making savory items like meats and sauces. Canola oil is a reasonable substitute when making milder or sweeter food items.

The best kind of olive oil for you, and perhaps not coincidentally the best-tasting, is extra-virgin cold-pressed oil from the first pressing. Cold-pressed oil is produced not by solvent extraction but by a mechanical process that preserves the chemical nature of the oil, the oil's flavor, and its natural antioxidants. If the label simply says "cold-pressed," this does not guarantee that it's from the first round of pressing. Extra-virgin olive oil is considered to be superior because it has the least acidity; virgin olive oil has slightly more acidity. Both types are mechanically extracted.

Have fun experimenting with different regions and brands to discover which flavors you like best. Personally, as I mentioned earlier, my favorite kind of olive oil is the kind that my relatives send me from Sicily; it has an unbelievable fruity, flowery flavor that I love. If you find olive oil to have too strong a flavor for you, take into account that the flavor of most olive oils greatly diminishes or disappears with cooking or baking. If it's still too strong, extra processing removes the aromatic substances that give olive oil its unique flavor, so you may prefer those types (usually called "light olive oil" or just "olive oil"); olive oil is more important for its fat content than nutrient content, so this type is perfectly acceptable.

Store your olive oil in a cool, dark place, preferably in an opaque bottle. Olive oil should last about a year or two if stored properly. Any oil will go rancid if stored for too long, so it's a good idea to smell oils before using them. Some brands add extra vitamin E to prevent oxidation and preserve their shelf life.

7. Consume a Moderate Amount of Low-Fat Dairy Products

Dairy in the traditional Mediterranean diet was mostly in the form of yogurt and cheese (especially feta)—since it was the only way to preserve milk in a hot climate where most people didn't have refrigerators. Because of this, when I was growing up in Sicily, our dairy intake was mostly in the form of cheese grated over pasta, and the only ones who drank milk were babies.

A healthy Mediterranean diet includes a moderate amount of dairy on a daily basis—**about 2 servings a day.** A serving constitutes 1 cup of skim milk or low-fat yogurt, or a 1-ounce portion of low-fat cheese.

Dairy foods are a good source of protein as well as calcium and vitamins A and D. Vitamin D helps the body to absorb calcium better so is sometimes added back to low-fat dairy products it's been removed from, as well as added to other products with calcium. The current calcium dietary recommendations for the average adult are around 1,000 to 1,300 mg per day, primarily to prevent osteoporosis, a bone-weakening condition affecting 10 million Americans, 80 percent of them women. Three times that number of people have osteopenia, or low bone mass, which precedes osteoporosis. There is some evidence to suggest that dairy products may also help prevent some types of cancer, but these studies are mixed and inconclusive at this time. Dairy consumption may offer a protective, if small, effect against heart disease, stroke, and diabetes, though again, studies are not in agreement. In the well-known DASH diet study, researchers saw large reductions in high blood pressure when the subjects added dairy products to a healthy diet. Adequate calcium consumption is especially important for children, adolescents, and pregnant women (for the developing fetus), as well as those over sixty years of age, when bone mass decreases significantly.

However, dairy foods can be very high in fat, especially harmful saturated fats, so reach for low-fat, part-skim, fat-free, or reduced-fat cheeses, milk, yogurt, ice cream, and the like. Calories are also significantly reduced in the lower-fat versions. For example, an 8-ounce glass of whole milk contains 150 calories, but the same amount of fat-free (skim) milk has only about 90. One ounce of regular cheddar cheese has 115 calories, whereas reduced-fat and low-fat varieties contain only 80 and 50, respectively. Be wary of low-fat ice creams and frozen yogurts, though, as sugar is often added to make up for the loss of flavor and texture that fat provides. And bear in mind that numerous plant foods are a great source of calcium: green leafy vegetables like kale and broccoli especially, as well as figs, almonds, sesame seeds, tofu, and beans.

YOGURT

In many parts of the Mediterranean, at least 1 cup of yogurt is eaten daily and is a major source of calcium in the diet. Yogurt is delicious alone, spooned over fruits or cereals, and mixed into dips or sauces.

CHEESE

In the Mediterranean, cheese is not eaten the way Americans eat it—slathered on pizza, burgers, and nachos. Rather, hard cheeses are lightly grated over pasta or vegetables, a small chunk of feta is crumbled into salads, a small serving of soft cheese might be mixed with vegetables, or a small amount of creamy cheese would be added to a dish for flavor.

Many cheeses contain a lot of fat, so they're neither low in calories nor heart-healthy. Hence, look for cheeses made from skim milk (it'll say so on the label), such as part-skim mozzarella. In fact, most cheeses come in reduced-fat versions these days and are a great way to enjoy the flavors you love at a much-reduced calorie load. If you love high-fat cheeses, such as muenster, cheddar, and goat, use them as added flavoring to salads or meals occasionally, as the Mediterraneans do. See the table below for a summary of the relative fat content in various cheeses.

FAT CONTENT OF VARIOUS CHEESES

Cheese (1 oz*)	Saturated Fat (g)	Total Fat (g)	Calories
Cream cheese, fat-free	0	0	27
Ricotta, fat-free	0	0	22
Ricotta, low-fat	1	1.6	30
Ricotta, part-skim	1.4	2.2	37
Ricotta, whole-milk	2.4	3.7	50
Cottage cheese (2% fat)	2.8	4	26
Mozzarella, part-skim	2.9	4.6	71
Mozzarella, whole-milk	3.7	6	80
Goat, soft	4	6	76
Feta	4.2	6	74
Neufchatel	4.2	6.5	73
Brie	4.9	8	95
Provolone	4.9	8	98
Edam	5	8	100
Gouda	5	8	100
Swiss	5	8	105
Monterey Jack	5	8.6	105
Gruyère	5.3	9	116
Blue cheese	5.3	8	99
Parmesan	5.4	7.5	130
Muenster	5.4	8.5	103
Fontina	5.4	8.7	109
Roquefort	5.5	8.5	103
American cheese	5.5	8.8	105
Colby	5.7	9.1	110
Cheddar	6	9.5	115

Cheese (1 oz*)	Saturated Fat (g)	Total Fat (g)	Calories
Cream cheese	6.2	9.9	99
Goat, hard	7	10	127

*An ounce isn't much—it's only about 1½ slices of processed cheese, a 1¼-inch cube of cheddar or most other hard cheeses, or the cheese on a small slice of pizza.

MILK

Milk is not consumed as a beverage in the traditional Mediterranean diet. Milk is a rich source of calcium, however, so I don't outlaw it. If you're going to get your dairy servings this way, stay away from whole milk—it has too many calories and too much saturated fat.

EGGS

Eggs were rarely eaten in my region when I was growing up, as no one could afford them; they were considered a real luxury. But you needn't fear them. Eggs are an inexpensive source of high-quality protein and a good source of vitamin B_{12}, vitamin E, riboflavin, niacin, iron, and phosphorus. Many people avoid them these days because of their association with high cholesterol. However, researcher Ancel Keys found in his studies that cholesterol in our diet seemed to be much less important in terms of promoting heart disease than saturated fat was. Thus, in regions that strictly followed a diet like the Mediterranean Prescription and also consumed a lot of eggs (sometimes at nearly every meal), heart attacks still remained a rarity. And modern research has confirmed his findings. So even though eggs contain a relatively large amount of cholesterol, four or fewer eggs per week is fine for a healthy adult (though there is no restriction on egg whites, since they are fat- and cholesterol-free).

For calorie cutting, instead of cooking up two eggs for yourself, try one yolk and two egg whites (about 100 calories). Decrease the number of yolks that you use for omelets, and add a variety of fresh vegetables. An egg breakfast may help you feel full longer, too. In one study of thirty overweight women who were given a breakfast of either a bagel, cream cheese, and yogurt (339 calories) or two eggs, toast, and jelly (340 calories), the egg group felt full longer and ate fewer calories both for lunch and dinner, and even the next day, when they could eat anything they liked.

IS THERE A LINK BETWEEN DAIRY CONSUMPTION AND WEIGHT LOSS?

There's been a great deal of press recently on the link between dairy food consumption and weight loss. This is a result of a number of studies that suggest calcium, especially calcium derived from dairy products, may help to regulate body fat. Much of this enthusiasm has been generated by the studies of Michael B. Zemel, from the University of Tennessee. In a headline-generating study funded by the National Dairy Council, where people went on either a control diet, a dairy-food-supplemented diet, or a calcium-pill-supplemented diet, all with the same number of calories, the last two groups lost more weight than the control group, with the most weight loss resulting from the diet with dairy foods. However, there were some important flaws to this study: it was the result of one small clinical trial consisting of thirty-two participants; it was a study of clinically obese participants, so the results can't be extrapolated for the nonobese; and the weight loss results from the dairy diet weren't dissimilar from what would be expected from the low-calorie diets they were on. Nevertheless, Dr. Zemel has published a multitude of self-referential papers supporting his claims, and the media has seized on his results, often misrepresenting them. You should know that in a review of twenty-six papers in which either calcium or dairy products were given in clinical trials without caloric restrictions, no weight loss occurred. In addition, studies in which dairy was added to the diets of normal-weight subjects did not demonstrate weight loss in the dairy users.

The pro-dairy hypothesis is not without other supporters, though, and it's possible there is something to it. Essentially, the jury is still out on whether dairy foods facilitate weight loss. It is my belief that while dairy may have a small effect on fat cell breakdown, it is nowhere *near* the benefits to health and weight loss to be found with following the guidelines of the Mediterranean Prescription on a day-to-day basis. The health benefits and weight-loss efficacy of the Mediterranean diet have been studied and confirmed for decades. Dairy may be an important component, but it is only one of twelve.

On the other hand, if you are substituting an 80-calorie low-fat yogurt for your daily Snickers candy bar (280 calories), you are most assuredly making a health-promoting, weight-loss-advancing decision! In this way, dairy products can absolutely help with weight loss, and I highly recommend them.

8. Eat Fish

Personally, this is my favorite part of the Mediterranean Prescription. I grew up on fish, and nowadays, I love to cook it, eat it, serve it to my friends and family, and teach others how to make a wonderfully light, delicious meal out of a fish and a few simple ingredients. My taste for it was born in Sicily. When I was growing up we weren't very far from the ocean, so the fish truck would come by every day. The vendor would yell out, "Fish! Fish for sale!" and they'd have their catch of the day on ice. My mother would call down from her balcony and ask, "What do you have today?" He'd tell her, and she'd tell him to give her a kilo of this and a kilo of that. She'd lower a wicker basket down on a rope, and the fish man would load the basket; she'd pull it up and then send it back down with money, so she'd never have to come downstairs. One of my pastimes was to go to the docks and get the fish right from the boats with my father and mother. Even today, whenever I go someplace new in the United States or abroad, I'll ask to be taken to the docks where the boats come in. If I'm staying in someone's home, I'll buy fish there and cook it up for my hosts.

One thing I would like to emphasize is that there is nothing like fresh fish. The standard freezing process can greatly alter fish's texture and flavor. This is why I eat fish like people all over the Mediterranean eat it—fresh from the market, never frozen—and strongly encourage you to do the same. If you can't get fresh fish, try to find fish that has been flash-frozen shortly after being caught. With advances in flash-freezing and shipping, great-tasting fish is available in more and more places across the country these days.

Many people associate fish with a healthy diet, as they should. However, once you have reached the Maintenance Stage, fish should be eaten in moderation compared to the Two-Week Weight Loss Stage, since the traditional Mediterranean diet was largely plant-based. Fish consumption in the Mediterranean in 1960 varied, mainly according to the proximity to the sea. For example, whereas we ate fish nearly every day, the Cretans only ate about 5 ounces of fish a week. Because it has been shown that a traditional Mediterranean health pattern can be found in people consuming much more than what the Cretans were eating, **I recommend eating fish up to eight times a week** (in 3- to 4-ounce portions) if you like. I encourage you to choose fish over chicken and red meat. Studies suggest that eating up to 40 ounces of fish a week can still maintain the benefit of the Mediterranean diet. However, bear in mind that the average adult needs only 50 to 60 grams of protein a day—most consume twice that. By following the Mediterranean Prescription, you can easily fulfill your daily protein needs eating much less meat than you're probably used to. When adhering to my advice and eating a salad before and two vegetables (or a vegetable and legume) with your meal, you will find yourself naturally cutting down on the amount of meat you eat. In fact, I typically eat a small dish of pasta, a small salad, and two vegetables along with my fish; if you eat like this, you will feel very full on 3 to 4 ounces of fish.

Fish is low in saturated fat, and in general it's a low-calorie, high-quality source of protein. Fatty fish such as salmon, mackerel, tuna, anchovies, trout, and herring are high in **omega-3 fatty acids,** which may reduce the risk of heart disease and stroke. They may also reduce the severity of asthma, rheumatoid arthritis, and other chronic inflammatory diseases. In one study, out of about two thousand men who'd recovered from a heart attack, the men who were counseled to increase their fatty fish intake had about 30 percent less risk of death from all causes over the course of two years. For these reasons, **I recommend that 2 to 3 servings of your fish intake per week be fatty fish, high in omega-3s.** In some studies, fish consumption is also associated with a reduction of fat around the abdomen (the "apple" body shape), which is the most harmful to your heart.

When I talk about fish, I am referring to the whole bounty of the Mediterranean Sea and beyond. My favorite Mediterranean fish aren't as widely known in America: try to find porgy, branzino, and orata at your local market, you won't be disappointed. Other favorites of mine are sardines, red snapper, and Spanish mackerel. Don't forget about shrimp, calamari, clams, mussels, lobster, and so on. Fish doesn't have to be an entrée, either; use it on salads and in soups, stews, and casseroles, as the Mediterraneans do. Try salmon, snapper, swordfish, tuna, haddock, halibut, or cod as substitutes for meat in your favorite beef recipes. As I note in my Two-Week Weight Loss Stage, the recipes don't have to be fancy or fussy: sauté, broil, bake, poach, steam, or grill your fresh fish or shellfish with a little olive oil, seasoning, and lemon, and serve!

9. Eat the Right Fats (Have a High Ratio of Unsaturated Fats to Saturated Fats in Your Diet)

While olive oil may be one of the pricier oils in the United States, in Sicily in the 1960s the cheapest and easiest fat to get was olive oil. Everyone grew olives and could get them pressed at the mill into olive oil. For flavoring they would sometimes get a little animal fat from the butcher—who in my town was my father—but meat itself was rarely eaten because most people couldn't afford it. This might have felt like deprivation to the grown-ups in my town, but it turned out to be an extraordinarily healthy combination for all of us. Olive oil is high in monounsaturated fat, the best kind of fat for your body. The fish we ate was rich in omega-3 fatty acids. The lack of red meat spared us from overindulging in harmful saturated fats. Nothing was processed either, of course, so we didn't have to worry about trans fats. Essentially, we had the perfect mix of dietary fat.

While the term *fat* has a negative association, in fact fats have many positive attributes. For one, fat improves the taste and texture of many foods. I'm sure it's no accident that we like them, since fats are also important for absorption of the fat-soluble vitamins A, D, E, and K, and they are important components of structures in our bodies such as muscles, nerves, membranes, and blood vessels. Our body needs fat because that is where energy is stored. Besides being the main source of energy for us, fat also cushions our organs and maintains body temperature. Furthermore, evidence suggests that a diet moderate in fat, versus a low-fat diet, is better for blood chemistry (it reduces triglycerides and improves cholesterol) and your cardiovascular disease risk profile.

Fat comes in three main forms: saturated, polyunsaturated (which includes omega-3 and omega-6 fats), and monounsaturated. While some fats are far better than others (see below), too much of any of these fats will increase cholesterol levels as well as body fat.

A QUICK PRIMER ON FAT TYPES, FROM BEST TO WORST

Monounsaturated Fat

The differences between types of fat are a result of the differences in their chemical structures. Fatty acids (the building blocks of fats) are combinations of mostly carbon and hydrogen atoms. A fatty acid that does not have the maximum possible number of hydrogen atoms attached to every carbon atom is called *unsaturated;* instead of bonding to hydrogen, one or more carbon atoms form a double bond with the next carbon. Monounsaturated fats have only one double bond per molecule. Because the double bond makes these molecules more unstable, the point at which it melts is lower, such that they're liquids even at room temperature. This liquid property of monounsaturated fats is very beneficial to the human body. You could think of it this way: which would be more likely to clog your drain, a liquid or a congealed concoction?

Monounsaturated fats are the best fats because they lower bad cholesterol (low-density lipoproteins, or LDL) without lowering good cholesterol (high-density lipoproteins, or HDL). What's more, **they may help you lose weight.** A recent small study published in the *British Journal of Nutrition* showed that on a diet of equal calories for four weeks, those consuming monounsaturated instead of saturated fats had a lower body weight and less fat mass at the conclusion of the study.

Oleic acid is a monounsaturated fat and the primary ***omega-9 fatty acid*** (fatty acids are classified by their chemical structure, and in the family of omega-9 fats, the first double bond is located on the ninth carbon atom). **Olive oil** is the monounsaturated all-star, as it consists of up to 80 percent oleic acid and may be a major reason why the Mediterranean diet is so good for you. Increased consumption of olive oil has been implicated in a reduction in cardiovascular disease, rheumatoid arthritis, and a variety of cancers; its intake has also has been shown to improve immune function, particularly the inflammatory processes associated with the immune system. In addition to olives, monounsaturated fats are concentrated in almonds, peanuts, pecans, cashews, hazelnuts, and macadamias (and their respective oils), as well as avocado.

Polyunsaturated Fat

Polyunsaturated fats have many double bonds between their carbon atoms. While this instability keeps them liquid at room temperature, just like monounsaturated fats, the increased instability is also likely why an oversupply of some of them can be deleterious to your health (see the discussion of omega-6 fatty acids below).

Polyunsaturated fats lower blood levels of the good kind of cholesterol, HDL, as well as the bad kind, LDL. Still, they benefit us because they keep the overall blood cholesterol down and decrease cholesterol deposits on artery walls. They may become toxic when used in deep-frying, though—another reason to avoid fried foods. When heated to high temperatures, the oils produce HNE (4-hydroxy-trans-2-nonenal), a highly toxic compound that's easily absorbed by the body. These compounds have been associated with a variety of illnesses, including cardiovascular disease, Parkinson's and Alzheimer's diseases, and liver problems.

Polyunsaturated fats are found in safflower, sesame, and sunflower seeds, corn and soybeans, and their oils.

Omega-3 fatty acids (also known as N-3 or ω-3 fatty acids) are a particular group of polyunsaturated fatty acids. Omega-3 fatty acids get their name because the first double bond is located on the third carbon atom. These polyunsaturated fatty acids are effective in helping protect against cardiovascular disease and cancer and in helping improve inflammatory processes.

The mechanisms through which omega-3 fatty acids may inhibit carcinogenesis, such as reducing immune-cell-mediated inflammation and inhibiting the growth and spread of tumors, are many and technical. Suffice it to say that omega-3 fatty acids appear to decrease your chance of getting cancer.

There is growing experimental evidence for the role of omega-3 fatty acids in reducing the risk of heart-related disorders such as coronary heart disease and sudden cardiac death. It is believed that they improve blood cholesterol levels and reduce blood clotting in vessel walls. Other major benefits are related to their role in the brain, which is largely made of the kind of fat that must be supplied by the diet. Omega-3 fats are essential for peak brain activity. Their beneficial properties have been studied in the treatment of a variety of mental conditions, such as depression, bipolar disorder, schizophrenia, Alzheimer's, chronic fatigue syndrome, and stress. Research has shown that essential fatty acids reduce the damage caused by high levels of stress hormones. Furthermore, there is strong evidence that omega-3 fats, including omega-3 fish oil supplements, can improve rheumatoid arthritis (and possibly osteoarthritis) symptoms such as pain, lack of strength, stiffness, and fatigue. There is some evidence that they may improve other autoimmune diseases as well, such as lupus.

Animal foods rich in omega-3 fatty acids include fatty fishes (the fattier the fish, the higher the omega-3 fatty acid content) such as salmon, halibut, mackerel, albacore (white) tuna, trout, anchovies, sardines, and herring. Foods that supply omega-3s to a lesser extent include shrimp, clams, yellowfin or bluefin (light) tuna, catfish, and cod.

Alpha-linolenic acid belongs to the group of omega-3 fatty acids but comes from plant sources such as green leafy vegetables, nuts, and seeds.

It is one of two essential fatty acids, called essential because they are not produced in our bodies but are necessary to maintaining health. Good sources are flaxseed and flaxseed oil, walnuts, canola oil, strawberries, kale, and soybeans. One of the most important aspects of the Mediterranean diet is that it is rich in both plant and animal sources of omega-3 fatty acids, particularly compared to the typical American diet.

Omega-6 fatty acids (also known as N-6 or ω-6 fatty acids) are another type of polyunsaturated fatty acid group that people need to consume to stay healthy. In the proper amounts, omega-6 fatty acids can help regulate inflammation and blood pressure as well as heart, gastrointestinal, and kidney functions. Omega-6s can help reduce the aches and pains of rheumatoid arthritis and relieve the discomforts of PMS, endometriosis, and fibrocystic breasts. They can reduce the symptoms of eczema, psoriasis, and probably other chronic skin conditions, such as acne and rosacea. They may also prevent and improve nerve damage in diabetics. Good dietary sources of omega-6 fatty acids include cereals, eggs, poultry, most vegetable oils, whole-grain breads, and trans-fat-free margarines.

Linoleic acid, an omega-6 fatty acid, is the second essential fatty acid, which the body cannot manufacture and so must be obtained from the diet. Sources of linoleic acid are vegetables, fruits, nuts, grains, seeds, and oils such as safflower, sunflower, corn, soya, pumpkin-seed, and wheat-germ.

A few of words of caution. Scientists are now finding that the health benefits of omega-6 fatty acids are present only when they are balanced properly. When we have too much polyunsaturated fat in our diet, it can promote inflammation, blood clotting, and possibly cancer cell growth. At the same time, these fats are necessary to our health since they include essential fatty acids. The **health problems arise when the ratio of omega-6 fat to omega-3 fat is too high.** Western diets range between 10:1 and 20:1 in favor of omega-6 fats, whereas the ideal ratio should only be about 3:1 or 4:1. By following the Mediterranean Prescription, you will keep the omega-6 fatty acids at a healthy proportion.

Saturated Fat

Let's get technical again here for a minute so that you understand what you're putting into your body when you eat saturated fats. As I've noted, all fatty acids (the building blocks of fat) are chains of mostly carbon and hydrogen atoms. A saturated fatty acid has the maximum possible number of hydrogen atoms attached to every carbon atom. It is therefore said to be "saturated" with hydrogen atoms. In addition, all of the carbons are attached to each other with single bonds—the most stable type of bond. Because of these stable bonds, the point at which saturated fats melt is higher—so at room temperature, these fats are solids (like butter, or the fat in meat). This stability also makes these fats a hazard in our bodies.

Of all the fats, saturated fat is the most potent determinant of high blood cholesterol levels. A high intake of saturated fats, like in the typical American diet, tends to keep the circulating LDL ("bad") cholesterol level high, which is related to heart disease, as I discussed before. Reducing your saturated fat intake and increasing the amount of unsaturated fat you eat is effective in lowering your LDL levels. Saturated fats are found in animal products, such as meat, poultry fat, butter, egg yolks, cream, ice cream, and whole milk, and also in tropical oils like coconut and palm oils.

Trans Fat

Trans fats are basically unsaturated fats that have been turned into saturated fats. The term *trans* refers to the fact that the hydrogen atoms attached to the carbon atoms are on opposite sides of the double bond (in nature, most molecules contain cis molecules, in which the hydrogens are on the same side of the bond). Though trans bonds can sometimes occur in trace amounts in nature in meat and dairy products (a result of fermentation in grazing animals), most have been created through a man-made process of adding hydrogen atoms, called hydrogenation. Unsaturated fats can be converted to saturated fats by hydrogenation; since this usually raises the melting point of the liquid fat and makes it a solid, the process is also called hardening. Manufacturers do this to increase the shelf life of the more unstable liquid fats, but, as you can guess, this turns a formerly healthy fat into one that has the same dangers as saturated fats.

Trans fatty acids increase LDL levels while decreasing HDL levels—the worst possible combination, as this raises the risk of coronary heart disease. Relative to saturated fat, trans fatty acids produce a lower total cholesterol level, but this is not necessarily a good thing, because our body needs higher amounts of HDL to be healthy.

While trans fats are certainly not healthy, their evils have been somewhat hyped in the media. They act in virtually the same way as saturated fats. The real problem has been that, though they do the same damage as saturated fats, until recently they were underreported on nutrition labels because the Food and Drug Administration didn't require them to be listed. This changed on January 1, 2006, and now food manufacturers are obliged to list the trans fat content on their products. Look for them on food labels, since they should be avoided, though no more so than saturated fats.

The most common trans fats are the hydrogenated fats found in processed foods such as margarines (stick more than tub), doughnuts, cookies, cakes, corn chips, potato chips, crackers, biscuits, muffins, dessert pies, dark breads, pastries, fried fish, french fries, and basically any product that contains partially hydrogenated oils. Look for the words *hydrogenated* or *partially hydrogenated* on the label; if you see them, you've got yourself a product with trans fats.

THE BIG FAT SUMMARY

Just by reading about the above fats, you can probably easily draw your own conclusions about which fats you should maximize and which you should minimize. Here is a rundown of my recommendations for the Mediterranean Prescription:

1. **Eat the right fats.** The message here is don't be afraid of fat, only worry about the bad kinds. While saturated and trans fats have clear health risks, **monounsaturated and polyunsaturated fats (especially omega-3s) are good for you**, are satisfying to eat, and help you feel full longer than carbohydrates. Despite the claims of many low-fat diets, much evidence exists that America's tremendous weight gain over the past several decades is *not* due to too much fat in the diet. For example, in 2004 the Centers for Disease Control reported that during the period from 1971 to the year 2000, the prevalence of obesity in the United States increased from 15 to 31 percent, while fat intake substantially *decreased* for both men and women ages twenty to seventy-four. In fact, **since the 1950s, fat consumption has *decreased*, while the percentage of the population that is overweight has *increased*.** The problem is that our total intake of calories has increased (mainly from carbohydrates).

2. **Have a high ratio of unsaturated fats to saturated fats in your diet.** Maximize monounsaturated fats and minimize saturated fats.

3. **Eat as high a ratio of omega-3 to omega-6 fats as you can.** Americans currently eat around ten to twenty times more

omega-6 fats compared to the amount of omega-3 fats they take in, instead of the recommended three to four times more.

4. **Use olive oil, in particular, in abundance**. It's a monounsaturated fat with copious health benefits.

5. **Avoid saturated fats as well as trans fats—they're equally bad for you.** This is where programs such as the Atkins diet fall short. While having a good percentage of fat in one's diet has consistently been shown to be part of a weight-reducing diet people can stick to, when that fat is saturated or trans, you risk creating a blood lipid profile that puts you at risk for heart disease and many other conditions. Read labels and skip products that contain saturated or hydrogenated fats.

6. **Getting your fat from nuts, seeds, and legumes gives you the added bonus of protein**. Since protein is even more satiating than fat, this combination should make you feel the fullest the longest (and avoids the saturated fats of red meat).

YOUR GUIDE TO CHOOSING HEALTHY FATS

The table below shows the range of fats, left to right, from best to worst. Food items often have more than one kind of fat in them, which is why there is some overlap. The table here tells you what the dominant fat is in each item to help you make healthy choices when selecting food.

GOOD			BAD	
Monounsaturated	**Polyunsaturated Omega-3**	**Polyunsaturated Omega-6**	**Saturated**	**Trans**
Olives, olive oil Flaxseeds, flaxseed oil Almonds Avocadoes Canola oil Peanuts, peanut oil	Flaxseed, flaxseed oil Canola oil Soybeans,** soybean oil** Walnuts, walnut oil Fish oil	Poultry Grapeseed oil Corn, corn oil Cottonseed oil Safflower oil Sesame oil Soybean oil**	Animal fat Cocoa butter Red meat Butter Dairy fat Coconut oil Palm or palm kernel oil	Hydrogenated or partially hydrogenated oils Shortening Cookies, cakes, doughnuts, pastries, and pies made with hydrogenated fats

GOOD			BAD	
Mono-unsaturated	**Poly-unsaturated Omega-3**	**Poly-unsaturated Omega-6**	**Saturated**	**Trans**
Many other nuts, such as pecans, cashews, hazelnuts, and macadamia nuts Margarine*	Mackerel Salmon Sardines Tuna Other fish Other nuts and seeds Margarine*	Sunflower oil Other oil-containing nuts and seeds Margarine*	Egg yolks Lard Margarine*	Fried food (fried in animal fat or hydrogenated fats) Margarine*

* Type of fat varies; check the label
** More omega-6 than omega-3

HIGH BLOOD CHOLESTEROL

High total and LDL cholesterol levels and low HDL cholesterol levels increase the risk of heart attack. The following table lists cholesterol levels and levels to shoot for. A total cholesterol measurement is the sum of all of the cholesterol in your blood. In general, the higher your total cholesterol, the greater your risk for heart disease. However, the ratio of HDL to LDL is more important than the total, since a high total could be the result of high HDL levels, which would be a good thing. HDL cholesterol is often referred to as the "good" cholesterol because it carries cholesterol in the blood away from other parts of the body back to the liver, which leads to its removal from the body; this helps keep cholesterol from building up on the walls of your arteries.

Measurement	Level of Cholesterol (mg/dL)	Level of Risk
	< 200	Desirable level; puts you at lower risk for heart disease
Total cholesterol	200–239	High
	>240	Dangerously high blood cholesterol; in general, a person with this level has more than twice the risk of heart disease compared to someone whose cholesterol is below 200
	< 40	A major risk factor for heart disease
HDL ("good") cholesterol	40–59	The higher your HDL, the better
	> 60	A measurement of 60 and above is considered protective against heart disease
	< 100	Optimal
LDL ("bad") cholesterol	100–129	Normal
	130–159	High
	> 160	Very High

I have had many of my patients go on cholesterol-reducing drugs for their high cholesterol. They often have the attitude that once they're on them, they can eat whatever they want. With this approach, however, they will be on these medications for the rest of their lives. It is far superior to reduce high cholesterol levels by losing weight, exercising, and eating a healthy diet, if possible. It's true that some people are genetically predisposed to have high cholesterol despite leading a healthy lifestyle; however, many people can control their cholesterol this way and live medication-free. What is most rewarding for me is to see my patients follow the Mediterranean Prescription and bring their high cholesterol levels down on their own.

10. *Engage in Regular Physical Activity*

When Ancel Keys followed the diets of populations around the globe, he came to the conclusion that nutrition was even more important than physical activity in terms of overall health. Nonetheless, the healthiest populations—those in the rural Mediterranean—typically labored long hours working their fields, tending their houses, making a living, and getting around. Indeed, in my Sicilian village forty years ago, only three families had cars. We didn't even have buses except to get from town to town. The closest we had to a cab was a donkey. This meant that to get anywhere, you pretty much had to walk. If you wanted to go to the beach, you walked. If you wanted to go to the playground, you walked. We worked hard, too. Everyone chipped in to tend the family's plot of land. Making a garden is demanding work—tilling the soil and removing the rocks, planting, irrigating, and harvesting. My mother worked from dawn until dusk fixing our family's meals and cleaning without the advantage of modern electrical appliances or "new and improved" cleaning solutions.

Regular exercise appears to increase longevity in both men and women, even if they only exercise once a week. It strengthens your bones and helps prevent osteoporosis. It also reduces the risk of coronary artery disease and heart attack by controlling blood cholesterol levels, decreasing the risk of obesity and diabetes, and lowering high blood pressure. Aerobic exercise in particular—exercise that gets your breathing and heart rates up, such as walking, jogging, and bicycle riding—builds endurance and increases the amount of oxygen-rich hemoglobin in your bloodstream, which helps the cardiovascular system to operate more efficiently. As a result, your body is better able to burn the fuel you consume in the form of fats and carbohydrates. Resistance exercises, such as weight lifting and repetitive pushing, pulling, and lifting exercises, on the other hand, primarily build muscle tissue and enhance your physical strength.

EXERCISE AND WEIGHT MAINTENANCE

In addition to exercise helping your heart, preventing disease, and developing your muscle tone, I am sure it comes as no surprise to you that being physically active helps you lose weight as well as maintain your new weight once the pounds are off. You can lose weight by following the Mediterranean Prescription without exercise, but you will find it much easier to achieve and maintain your ideal weight with exercise. We'll talk more about exercise as an aid to weight loss later. As for maintaining your weight with exercise, the fact of the matter is that studies show over and over that few people can maintain substantial weight loss without continued physical activity. Indeed, physical activity stands out as one of the best predictors of long-term success in weight reduction.

As you probably noticed, your body is remarkably efficient at maintaining a steady weight. Our body weight stays relatively constant over time unless radical changes occur in our lives. Like a thermostat, the central nervous system uses both chemical and psychological feedback to maintain constant levels of lean body mass (muscle) and fat over time. This process happens in spite of significant temporary changes such as transient dieting and short-term exercise programs. When the diet or exercise program ends, both lean and fat body mass generally return to the starting level. Herein lies the key to why the Mediterranean Prescription is a prescription for life: **short-term diets don't keep the weight off forever**—your eating and exercise habits need to fundamentally change to resist the powerful drives of your body to restore it to its previous weight. The good news is, you can still eat delicious, filling food, and changing just requires a painless readjustment of your habits.

CHANGING YOUR SET POINT

If you've been at a certain weight for quite a while, this weight is probably your current established set point, or the weight your body is trying to maintain. Your metabolic rate—the rate at which you burn calories—will thus tend to speed up and burn more calories if you've eaten more than your normal amount and, alas, will tend to slow down when you eat less than normal, all to maintain this steady weight. Because your metabolic rate will decelerate as a result of weight loss, exercise should be employed to compensate for this.

When you lose weight at a fast rate, you will burn muscle tissue as well as fat, which adds to the slowdown of your metabolic rate. Your metabolic rate increases with lean body mass, so activities that build and tone muscle will burn more calories, allowing you to either lose weight, eat more than you're accustomed to without gaining weight, or maintain your current weight even if it's at a slower metabolic rate.

Taking up the Mediterranean Prescription as a lifestyle will stabilize your nutritional intake and keep you active. After a while the starvation alarm bells from the weight loss will stop going off in your body, and your set point should settle down at a lower weight. At this time you'll be able to scale back the amount of exercise you do. A patient of mine from a few years ago is a perfect example. She dieted and worked out at a gym for an hour a day for about three months straight while she lost thirty pounds. After a while, she only required two to three days a week at the gym to maintain her trim figure. Personally, I take the stairs whenever I can, walk to do my errands as much as time permits, and go to the gym four times a week for forty to forty-five minutes each time. This is the regimen that works for me to maintain my weight. Trial and error will guide you to the amount of exercise you require to maintain your weight loss, which is a very personal formula.

PRECAUTIONS

If you have health problems, it is best to consult your physician to find out which activities are safe for you. Some conditions such as arthritis can be very painful, but low-impact exercising such as swimming or walking might be possible. Don't assume that exercise is prohibited for your condition, because it may actually improve it. If you are quite overweight and have been sedentary for a long time, I strongly encourage you to have a physical exam by your doctor and talk to him or her about an exercise program before you begin.

GENERAL RECOMMENDATIONS

It is outside the scope of this book to prescribe specific exercise regimens, but I'd like to give you some general principles.

My most important advice is to make time in your routine for exercise. Exercise is unquestionably a **time commitment** in what is a busy world for most of us. What I try to convey to my patients is that they consider the sacrifice versus the payoff: a handful of hours out of our week exercising makes us feel healthier, younger, stronger, more energetic, and more attractive. It improves our mood, enhances our self-esteem and psychological well-being, decreases stress and anxiety, and improves our sex life in terms of libido, potency, stimulation, and satisfaction. In other words, the time you devote to exercise makes *all* the rest of your waking hours a far more enjoyable place to be.

Current national guidelines suggest that a **minimum of 150 minutes a week** (or about thirty minutes a day, five days a week) of exercise is necessary to improve health. However, some studies suggest that a more vigorous routine is necessary to prevent weight regain in previously overweight and obese individuals, such as **200 to 300 minutes per week or more.** Try to begin with 150 minutes a week, and progress from there. Aspire to get up to an hour of slow walking or half an hour of moderate or brisk walking a day, or three and a half to five miles of brisk walking every day, depending on your needs.

The above recommendations are based on walking. The more vigorously you exercise, the less time you can spend doing it. You burn more calories the harder you work: for example, you burn around four calories a minute for slower activities such as walking, slow dancing, and gardening; seven calories per minute for fast walking, aerobics, light weight lifting, and moderate activity on a piece of exercise equipment; and ten calories per minute for vigorous activity like running, swimming laps, and heavy weight lifting.

While a daily fifteen-minute walk or other small increases in daily exercise may not be enough to prevent obesity, if you've previously been sedentary they are important steps to easing into a more active life. **If it's all you can manage, start out with one fifteen-minute walk a day, and add on more as you are able.** Try dividing thirty to forty minutes of exercise per day into several ten-minute bouts of exercise. Eventually, you will establish the amount of exercise necessary to stabilize your body weight. If you feel as if you are gaining weight, increase your amount of aerobic exercise, such as brisk walking, jogging, hiking, swimming, aerobics, or cycling.

Resistance Training

Irrespective of dieting, inactive people lose about 10 percent of their muscle mass every ten years after the age of twenty-five. However, with regular resistance training it is possible to regain this muscle mass. Although it's not generally as effective as aerobic training for burning calories, resistance training will still raise one's metabolic rate.

Keep Moving: The Benefits of Fidgeting

Recently scientists at the Mayo Clinic reported a striking difference in non-exercise activity levels between lean and overweight people. Overweight subjects tended to sit, while the lean ones were more restless and spent a total of two more hours a day on their feet, standing, pacing around, and fidgeting. The difference translated into a startling 350 calories a day—enough for the overweight people to take off thirty to forty pounds a year if they would get moving.

Don't Calculate Calories

I do *not* recommend calculating how much you eat versus how much exercise you need to do to burn it off. As with my diet plan, I firmly believe that simplicity is the key to the implementation of any fitness plan, and the formula for calories in versus calories burned is just too complicated, as it depends on many factors, such as your muscle mass, fat mass, and the other components of your diet, which are constantly in flux. Rather, eat healthily by following the guidelines in the Mediterranean Prescription, and exercise regularly. Continually tweak the amount of exercise you do each week by paying attention to your body: if your pants are getting a little tight, add an extra run that week, or if they are getting too loose, take some time off and relax!

Turn Off the TV

It has been said that the single greatest behavioral predictor of obesity in children and adults is the amount of television viewing. The relationship is nearly as strong as what you see between smoking and lung cancer. Contrary to what you might think, it's estimated that only about a third of the effect comes from the hours of sedentary viewing—the other two-thirds is the effect of advertising nudging us to feel like eating and coaxing us into making unwholesome food choices when we're away from the television.

KIDS AND EXERCISE

The three most important reasons for encouraging your children to be physically active and get exercise on a regular basis are (1) to support healthy habits that they will retain throughout their lives, (2) to prevent childhood overweight and obesity, and (3) to promote healthy, strong bone development. Teaching kids to be active is a lesson that will enhance their health and their quality of life their entire lives. The best lesson for them is leading by parental example!

Childhood overweight and obesity can be very unhealthy and cause the development of weight-related diseases commonly seen in adults, such as diabetes. The effects of obesity on cardiovascular health can begin in childhood as well, increasing the risk of developing coronary artery disease as an adult. Even if overweight young people do achieve a normal weight later in life, statistics show that obesity in the first twenty years of life significantly increases death rates once they become adults over age fifty. Furthermore, being overweight as a child can set the stage for becoming an overweight or obese adult, as it is a significant predictor for adult overweight and obesity. Obese adults who were obese as children may also have less success in weight reduction programs, so they need to be extra diligent to achieve weight loss. And not to be overlooked is that being an overweight child can be quite emotionally painful, as much as or more so than it is for adults.

Bone development for kids is crucial because there is only one window for accumulating bone mass: the first two decades of life. Peak bone mass is acheived by the end of adolescence, and we steadily lose bone mass thereafter. As kids are growing up, they can build robust bones by being physically active (in addition to having a diet rich in calcium). If kids are sedentary, they don't grow as much bone mass, and as they lose bone mass as adults, they can eventually develop osteoporosis.

Talk to your pediatrician about healthful levels of exercise for your children.

Suggestions to Squeeze More Activity into Your Day

- **Take the stairs** instead of the elevator, especially if the distance is three floors or less.
- **Park farther away** from where you're going so you have to walk more to get there and back.
- **Get off the bus or train** a stop or two early and walk the rest of the way.
- **Walk, roller-skate, or ride your bike to work** and back if the distance is reasonable.
- **Join a gym.** You'll be a lot more likely to make the time for exercise if you're paying a monthly fee. Furthermore, the peer pressure of the

others at the gym is much more effective than a home-exercise routine in terms of exertion and time spent exercising.

- **Take exercise classes**.
- **Get home-exercise equipment** and/or entertaining exercise videos if joining a gym is not an option or if you feel too self-conscious about your appearance to go to a public gym.
- **Start your day with an early morning walk, jog, or workout.** This eliminates procrastination techniques you may come up with throughout the day, and leaves evening time to spend with your friends or family.
- **Have your walk, jog, or workout directly after work** if you have more energy at the end of the day; not stopping home first prevents inertia from foiling your best intentions to exercise.
- **Use your lunch break for a walk or quick workout**; you'll likely find yourself more energized than you would be after a heavy lunch.
- **Get an exercise partner**; you'll be much less likely to cancel your exercise commitment if you're accountable to someone, in addition to it making your exercise more enjoyable.
- **Join a club** for walkers, joggers, runners, bikers, hikers, swimmers, tennis players, golfers, and so on, or start one!
- **Play actively with your kids or dog**; it'll be good for them, too.
- **Turn off the TV** and take a walk! Limit TV and video-game time for kids as well (no more than two hours a day). One of the most reliable predictors of obesity is how much television a person watches . . . need I say more?
- **Place a treadmill in front of the TV** if you can't kick your *Law and Order* habit, and exercise while you watch; or exercise during the commercials with sit-ups, leg lifts, push-ups, and the like.

11. Drink Wine (Especially Red) in Moderation, if You Choose

Every year in Sicily, my family would go into the country, harvest grapes together, and make our own wine, which we would then drink throughout the year. We always had a taste of wine with our meals. We began drinking it, diluted with water, even as children (not that I am recommending this, but that was our tradition). We'd often make a sangria with wine and fresh fruit. We would marinate pears, peaches, apples, and other fruits, which took on the flavor of the wine—delicious! Even the kids would get the fruit pieces to taste.

Drinking wine is a long-standing, popular tradition in the Mediterranean and is often included in descriptions of a healthy Mediterranean diet, which is supported by numerous research papers. There are some important potential negative aspects you should be aware of, however, which is why it is the only component of the Mediterranean Prescription in which I leave its consumption completely up to you.

TO YOUR HEALTH

First, the benefits. Moderate consumption of red wine has been associated with lowering the risk of developing coronary heart disease. Since oxidation is believed to be a central mechanism for the development of heart disease, the polyphenol antioxidants found in wine are likely candidates for its protective effect. To get technical, the abundant polyphenols found in red wine are anthocyanosides (flavonoids that provide color to the skins of red and black grapes), quercetin, proanthocyanidins (a group of tannins), catechins, stilbenes, and other phenolics. These antioxidants are also thought to be responsible for increasing HDL cholesterol, moderately reducing LDL cholesterol, helping prevent atherosclerosis, reducing the incidence of ischemic stroke (stroke caused by blood clots), and suppressing certain kinds of cancer cell growth. There is also evidence that suggests red wine may help reduce high blood pressure, reduce incidence of heart attacks, reduce development of peptic ulcers, lower incidence of gallstones and kidney stones, diminish occurrence of age-related macular degeneration (the most common cause of blindness in adults over sixty-five), preserve bone density, improve insulin resistance (which could lead to diabetes), and inhibit clot formation (similar to the effects of aspirin). It has also been related to a decreased susceptibility to colds.

Epidemiological studies repeatedly show that middle-aged men and women who regularly drink a moderate amount of alcohol have lower death rates from all causes in comparison with both abstainers and heavy drinkers. For example, in a recent study of about fifteen hundred Italian men, moderate drinkers (mostly red wine drinkers) had two extra years of life expectancy when compared to occasional and heavy drinkers.

CONSIDERATIONS AND RECOMMENDATIONS

Nevertheless, there are some important caveats to consider with alcohol. I do not advocate the consumption of alcoholic beverages for pregnant women, people who are prone to addiction, those who are taking medication that adversely interacts with alcohol, those with religious reasons for abstaining, or people who have unpleasant reactions to drinking. Furthermore, there are some general health risks associated with the consumption of alcohol. Certain cancers appear to be more prevalent in alcohol drinkers, mostly related to the upper digestive tract: oral cavity, larynx, esophageal, and liver cancer. In addition, the combination of tobacco and alcohol increases the tumor-producing effects of tobacco by 40 to 280 percent (though this effect appears to be stronger for spirits and beer than it is for wine). Alcohol consumption may also increase the risk for breast cancer, although reports are inconsistent, and some have even found that moderate consumption slightly decreases the risk. Alcohol may also increase the risk of hemorrhagic strokes (strokes that result from bleeding in the brain). Other potential health consequences of regular alcohol consumption include hypertension, liver disease, and violent and accidental death.

The key to alcohol consumption may be moderation. The maximum health benefits to be gained from red wine consumption appear to occur within a range of **1 to 2 glasses per day,** which is what I recommend. If you choose to follow the Mediterranean tradition and have a glass or two of red wine a day, be aware that the Mediterraneans, past and present, largely tend to take theirs with their meals. I would argue that that would be the most enjoyable time to have your glass of wine, and it just may be the healthiest time as well.

12. *Eat Only Small Amounts of Red Meat and Meat Products*

The Mediterranean region doesn't produce much beef, since the rocky terrain and limited pastureland are unsuited for cattle. Around the time Ancel Keys was doing his initial Mediterranean diet studies, most peo-

ple couldn't afford much meat of any kind anyway. Of red meat, they only ate veal (young cattle) and lamb once in a while. They would most often use it as a small part of a meal rather than as the center, or they would have it on a special occasion or holiday. This is very similar to the way I grew up in Sicily. In my youth, we ate more red meat than other families because my father happened to be a butcher, but we were the exception, and even then, we ate it only rarely. Meals mainly consisted of pasta, vegetables, legumes, and fish. We also had chicken regularly since everyone used to raise their own chickens. We'd have lamb occasionally, too, especially during the holidays.

The Italians and other Mediterraneans thus were accidental examples of how eating very little red meat could be beneficial to health. Over time, the richer these populations grew, the more meat they consumed . . . and the more heart disease, diabetes, and cancer they developed as well.

High consumption of red meat is strongly linked to the development of heart disease. Given that cardiovascular disease is the number one killer of both men and women in the United States, this should not be taken lightly. The reason red meat is connected to heart disease is because it is the main source of saturated fat in a typical Western diet (mostly from beef and pork). Saturated fat elevates LDL ("bad") cholesterol and the risk of arterial blockage, as I've already noted. Red meat and processed meat have also been shown to increase the incidence of **type 2 diabetes;** the mechanism is not entirely known, but it is believed to be related to their high saturated fat content (likely the major factor), as well as nitrites (used in processed meats as a preservative), heme iron (the iron found in meat), and their contribution to high caloric intake. Furthermore, excessive consumption of red meat may increase the risk of **colorectal cancer.**

It's important to remember that the saturated fat in red meat isn't just bad for your health; it also translates into **higher calories compared to lower-fat meats.** While 3 ounces of porterhouse steak, ground beef, and sirloin are 300, 250, and 165 calories, respectively, the same amount of chicken, fish (e.g., cod), and shellfish (e.g., Alaskan king crab) are about 140, 90, and 80 calories, respectively. Examine the table below to see the correlation between the amount of fat and calories among different meats.

FAT AND CALORIES IN VARIOUS KINDS OF MEAT

Meat Type (3 oz)	Saturated Fat (g)	Total Fat (g)	Calories
Steak, porterhouse	10	23	300
Chicken, light meat, fried w/ skin	5*	15	277
Lamb, loin	9	20	263
Hamburger	7	17	248
Tenderloin	7	17	247
Hamburger, extra-lean	5	13	225
Pork, loin	3	8	178
Lamb, leg, lean	2	7	162
Chicken, dark meat, skinless	2	6.1	159
Tuna, fresh bluefin	1.4	5	156
Ham	3	8	151
Veal, loin	6	2	149
Chicken, light meat, skinless	1.1	3.8	147
Turkey, light meat, no skin	0.9	2.7	134
Salmon	0.6	4	127
Ham, extra-lean	2	5	123
Halibut	0.3	2.5	119
Tuna, white, canned in water	0.7	2.5	109
Snapper	0.3	1.5	109
Cod	0.1	0.7	90

* Depends on the kind of oil it's cooked in

The United States is firmly entrenched in the meat-as-main-course mentality. The first national daily dietary guidelines, publicized in the 1940s by the United States Department of Agriculture (USDA), were aimed primarily at correcting nutritional deficiencies. The USDA included nutritional guidelines to help people deal with the shortage of food supplies during World War II. Thus, people were educated to believe that meat, potatoes, a slice of buttered white bread, and a big glass of milk was the healthiest meal around (it provided protein, iron, calcium, and no shortage of calories). The recommendations evolved somewhat over the years, but the idea persists in many people's minds that a good-size portion of meat should be the star of a proper, healthy meal. The problem is, we now know that this isn't the case.

The USDA has not done a perfect job in communicating this information. It doesn't help that the national dietary health recommendations—now the famous food pyramid—are published by the United States Department of Agriculture, not the National Institutes of Health or the Department of Health and Human Services, departments charged with promoting health. The USDA's primary job is to promote and regulate the commerce of agriculture; its pyramids are the focus of intense lobbying by, among others, the sugar, dairy, cereal, and meat industries. Though the latest pyramid is clearly headed in the right direction, it is not the strict outcome of vast comparative nutritional studies, such as the Mediterranean diet was born of. That's something to think about the next time you are trying to decide between the steak and the pasta primavera.

Lean meat is allowed in the Mediterranean Prescription one to two times a week. This could be 3 to 4 ounces of lean veal, lean pork, or other lean red meat (meats with the words *loin* or *round* in them usually have the lowest fat). As for high-saturated-fat red meats, like porterhouse steak and hamburger, I recommend you keep them to a minimum, such as a once-a-month splurge, if any.

WHAT ABOUT POULTRY?

While poultry was not consumed in abundance in the traditional Mediterranean diet, it can be a healthy part of your diet. The key is how you eat it and how much you eat. As you can see from the table above, the light and dark parts of poultry are not equal in terms of saturated fat content or calorie count. For this reason, when you are eating poultry, choose the leaner, lighter cuts. In some of my recipes I instruct you to cook chicken pieces with the skin on, but this is only for flavor. Poultry skin has a layer of fat to it and should always be removed before eating. If you want to further minimize animal fat in your diet and don't want the fat of the skin to be absorbed into the chicken, remove the skin prior to cooking as well. My mother takes the skin off chicken and then boils the meat before she bakes it; this preserves the moistness. Poultry should be broiled, roasted, poached, or grilled, never fried (unless you're sautéing it in a little olive oil). **I allow chicken (or other light, skinless poultry) one to two times a week during the Maintenance Stage.** As with any meat, fill up on grains, vegetables, and legumes so you keep the portion sizes of the poultry down (e.g., 3 to 4 ounces), or eat it as an addition to salads, soups, and pastas instead of as the main attraction.

MINIMIZING RED MEAT

Strive to cut down on the meat portion of your meals little by little. Make more vegetables per meal, and rather than putting the serving dishes on the table, try plating your meals in the kitchen, serving a larger vegetable portion and smaller meat portion than usual. (See the section on vegetables for more ideas on reducing meat intake.) If weight loss isn't a concern, increase grains and legumes as well. By increasing the protein and volume of other foods, you won't miss the place where red meat used to be. In my home, fish or meat is always accompanied by two vegetables and a salad and preceded by a small dish of pasta. By the time you get to the entrée, you will only require a small serving, as you are probably already full.

Summary: The Whole Is Greater than the Parts

It's important to remember that the above dietary components of the Mediterranean Prescription find their magnificent benefit when taken together. Many studies suggest that singling out an element here or there is not sufficient. Scientists don't quite know why yet. For example, one of the largest Mediterranean diet studies was published in the *New England Journal of Medicine* in 2003, in which over twenty-two thousand men were studied for three and a half years. It showed that despite a robust association between the overall Mediterranean diet and decreased death rate, no appreciable associations were seen for most of the *individual* components of the Mediterranean diet. Another study, published in 2005 in the *Journal of Nutrition*, demonstrated that men consuming *either* low amounts of saturated fat *or* high amounts of fruits and vegetables did not have a significantly lower risk of mortality; however, those who did *both* had about a 65 percent lower risk of death from coronary heart disease.

It should be further pointed out that the antioxidants and micronutrients that we believe to be the beneficial components of the Mediterranean diet have been shown to be by far the most effective in their original form—in nature's fruits, vegetables, legumes, nuts, and seeds; grains as close to their natural state as possible; olive oil in its purest form; dairy products; red wine; and fresh fish from our lakes, oceans, and seas—

rather than in pill form. Some micronutrient supplements may even be harmful, especially if taken in too high a dosage. Essentially, at this time we know of no shortcut or substitute to achieve the health benefits you will reap from following the full Mediterranean Prescription.

THE MEDITERRANEAN LIFESTYLE: *What It Is and Why It's Good for You*

EVERY SUNDAY AT MY GRANDMOTHER'S HOUSE WHEN I WAS GROWING UP, fifteen or twenty of my family members and I would gather for an early afternoon dinner. Every weekday, my brother and I would come home from school to eat lunch with my immediate family, and we would reconvene at dinnertime. On weekends, we'd often go to the country for the day with my extended family and friends to relax and cook together. Everyone knew everyone else—we knew when someone was born or fell sick or died, and we went through life together as a community of people who cared about each other.

In the Mediterranean, staying active, unwinding, enjoying time with family and friends, and appreciating good food are all considered important to a successful life, and indeed, it turns out that the elements of this lifestyle contribute to good health as well. When the studies on Mediterranean eating habits began, especially before the 1960s, the Mediterranean lifestyle differed significantly from today's modern Western one. Because the activities of daily living required physical labor, the people easily achieved far higher levels of exercise than most people in our society do today. Their lives may have been less stressed. Family and community ties were quite strong. People came together for unhurried meals and took midafternoon rests before returning to the physical labors required to earn a living. This isn't to say that life was easy, just that priorities and demands were different. Current research indicates that exercise, stress reduction, and strong social support help reduce the risk of heart disease and many other chronic diseases. The traditional Mediterranean lifestyle combined all of these elements and probably contributed significantly to the good health of the region.

While **physical activity can be increased** (see my section on exercise in chapter 1), dealing with stress is trickier, though not to be overlooked. **Stress has physical consequences.** The adrenaline rush from stress raises levels of a hormone called cortisol. If stress continues, elevated cortisol levels over time can cause depression of the immune system, clumping of blood platelets (which can increase the risk of heart attack), bone loss, and increased insulin production. In traditional Mediterranean culture, people had many mechanisms for dealing with stress. Family bonds were strong and of the utmost importance. The community support network was broad, and friends and neighbors supported each other. I would encourage you to seek out this same support for yourself, even if you live in a large, seemingly alienating metropolis. Find clubs that share your interests, join a religious organization, organize get-togethers with your friends, and of course spend time with your family.

Make it a goal to share at least one meal a day with friends or family. In the Mediterranean, spending time with family is a priority and is often centered around a meal. Preparation of the meal is equally important and can be a fun activity for the whole family. Many of us don't have the time in our day that the Mediterraneans spent making and eating their meals, but we can probably squeeze a little more time from our day for relaxing and enjoying food and family. One easy step toward this end is to involve the whole family in food preparation rather than having just one cook in the kitchen. It can be a wonderful time to teach and learn and spend time together. I greatly encourage you to resist the fast-food lifestyle and to embrace the Italian tradition of good food as a focal point, where mealtime is a time to enjoy, gather, and linger. Get the freshest ingredients you can and sample delicious recipes. **Food should be a pleasure,** not fraught with stress, guilt, and anxiety.

Italians epitomize this way of thinking: they live for food. They think about it a lot, they plan around it, they spend a lot of time preparing it, and they devote a lot of time to savoring and enjoying it. Let me give you an example of how important it is to Italians. I was treating an older southern Italian man with many ailments, and his extended family was very involved in his care. At one point I had to tell them, "Your father is a diabetic." Later I had to tell them, "Because of complications owing to the diabetes, your father needs an amputation." And then I had to tell them, "Your father is going to require open heart surgery because he has heart disease." Each time the news was received as well as could be expected, with no discussion from anyone. Then one day I had to tell them, "Your father needs a routine colonoscopy, so he can't eat anything from the evening until the next afternoon, when he gets the procedure." All of a sudden, after the family was told he couldn't eat, everyone was up in arms, and I got calls from ten frantic relatives yelling into the phone. "He can't eat? What do you mean he can't eat? Why can't he eat? Is he that sick?" In their minds, if a person can eat, he must be healthy, and if he can't, something must be gravely wrong. Everything relates back to food.

Recently scientists have been coming up with compelling reasons for families to pay attention to mealtime and pull up a chair around the dining room table. In the last few years studies have shown that, among preadolescent and adolescent kids, more frequent meals with the family were associated with a lower risk of smoking, drinking, and marijuana use; a lower risk of depressive symptoms and suicidal thoughts; less sexual activity; and fewer eating disorders. Furthermore, family meals encourage vocabulary growth in younger children and are associated with better grades. Regular family meals also provide an opportunity to establish a sense of belonging to a family unit and provide an important time for families to be together and talk, having time together that's not stressful, enjoying each other's company, and being around food. A handful of studies have also suggested that eating as a family improves children's consumption of fruits and vegetables, grains, fiber, and vitamins and minerals. Children who have family meals also eat less fried food, saturated fat, and soda. You obviously can further this trend by making healthy family dinner selections and leading by example.

Unfortunately, according to several surveys, 30 to 40 percent of families do not eat dinner together. **Many families that do dine together make a concerted effort to carve out the time.** My family made it the utmost priority for all of us to eat together. For example, when I was a kid, I couldn't play Little League baseball because I had to be home for dinner with the family at 1:30 on Sundays, when the games were held. I didn't understand at the time why I couldn't play baseball, but in retrospect I am so grateful for my family's commitment. This was our culture, and now studies show the benefits.

THE HEALTH BENEFITS OF THE MEDITERRANEAN PRESCRIPTION: *Living Healthier and Longer*

In the United States, as well as most other industrialized countries, cardiovascular disease and cancer are ranked as the top two leading causes of death, and together account for nearly half of all deaths. Indeed, it'd be hard to find someone who didn't have a case in their family or in someone's close to them. Worldwide, the numbers are so large they're numbing: cardiovascular disease accounts for around seventeen million deaths (about 30 percent of the total), while cancer contributes to approximately seven million deaths (about 13 percent). The amazing thing is that both are strongly linked to *lifestyle choices*—one of the most important of which is diet. For example, it has been estimated that around one-third of all cancer deaths in the United States could be avoided simply through dietary modification. A 2005 World Health Organization report stated that up to 2.6 million deaths worldwide and 31 percent of cardiovascular disease may be attributed simply to inadequate consumption of fruits and vegetables.

As I have said earlier, the Mediterranean diet has been studied since the 1950s, and the region stood out in worldwide nutritional research that showed its inhabitants were the healthiest, with the least heart disease and the longest life spans. Since that time, a great deal of research has been carried out to expand on the many healthful effects of the diet, more of which we're finding out every day. Some of the numerous diseases and conditions that can be potentially prevented or improved by following the Mediterranean diet are:

- Obesity
- Cardiovascular disease
- Heart attack
- Cancer
- Arthritis
- Type 2 diabetes
- Hypertension
- Metabolic syndrome

In addition to the Mediterranean lifestyle helping people achieve a healthy weight and level of physical activity, it is believed that the Mediterranean diet's mix of antioxidants, phytochemicals, monounsaturated fats, omega-3 fatty acids, and fiber is the key to its health-promoting qualities. Food intake produces oxidation, which leads to a state that promotes inflammation. Inflammation on a very fundamental level—such as in your arteries—may lead to a variety of illnesses. One of the leading theories of the mechanism behind the diet's protective effects is that its components prevent this inflammation, which is a common link among many of the conditions the diet improves or prevents. More research needs to be done to explain the exact workings, but in the meantime, it's important to know that there is convincing evidence that a number of illnesses can be reduced in severity or avoided just by changing your eating habits, with no drug or surgical intervention whatsoever. If any of these conditions run in your family, this advice should be considered even more seriously, since this puts you at greater risk already.

Obesity

Many studies have confirmed the successful long-term use of the Mediterranean diet in weight loss. One research group even stated, "Long-term follow-up of this diet program is at least as effective as any diet or diet-and-drug therapy published." In a diet review paper, after criticizing other restrictive diets, one obesity expert affirmed that "the Mediterranean diet was ideal, better tasting, proven heart-protective, with increased longevity." The most common statements in the medical literature relate to its capacity for long-term participation and adherence, in addition to the many health benefits it bestows.

Heart Disease

The relationship between the Mediterranean diet and heart disease is likely the most studied aspect of the diet. The diet has a remarkable ability to protect your heart. Perhaps most important is its capacity to reduce the risk factors for cardiovascular disease, such as increased body weight, high blood pressure, and high LDL and low HDL cholesterol. Countless studies have shown its protective effects against cardiovascular disease, atherosclerosis, and heart attack. One example is the Lyon Diet Heart Study, in which participants on the Mediterranean diet were shown to have a nearly 70 percent reduction in risk of coronary events (such as heart attack) and cardiac deaths. In another study, Harvard researchers determined that by replacing 5 percent of daily saturated fat with unsaturated fat, a woman's risk for heart disease could be reduced by 42 percent. An important aspect the heart researchers brought up repeatedly was the participants' terrific propensity to adhere to the diet: in one of the longest studies, patients were still closely following the Mediterranean diet recommended to them after four years. Low-fat diets, which are also recommended for a healthy heart, tend to be much harder for people to stick to.

Cancer

The incidence of cancer overall in Mediterranean countries is lower than in the United States, the United Kingdom, and Scandinavian countries. Mortality statistics from the World Health Organization, as well as epidemiological studies, have clearly documented the low incidence of most cancers and the long survival of people in the Mediterranean, even despite a high prevalence of smoking. Migrant studies have shown that when people move out of Mediterranean regions and their diets change, the protective effect doesn't hold, so it does not appear to be genetic. Rather, the effects are believed to come from a combination of factors: high unsaturated fat intake, low saturated fat consumption, high antioxidants, oleic acid (from olive oil), high consumption of omega-3 fatty acids, relatively low intake of omega-6 fats, and fiber. Inflammatory as well as immune factors appear to be at least partially responsible for cancer development, and the combined elements of the Mediterranean diet may counteract that. (Of note is that most of the studies testing the effect of one single dietary factor on cancer risk have been disappointing.)

Although estimates are crude, it can be calculated that up to 25 percent of the incidence of colorectal cancer, 15 percent of breast cancer cases, and 10 percent of cases of prostate, pancreatic, and endometrial cancer could be prevented if developed Western countries adopted the Mediterranean way of eating. The Mediterranean diet also favorably affects the risk of upper airway and digestive tract cancers, such as mouth, pharynx, esophagus, and larynx. High fruit and vegetable intake alone appears to help reduce cancers of the mouth, esophagus, stomach, large bowel, liver, pancreas, larynx, lung, breast, endometrium, cervix, prostate, bladder, and kidney.

Arthritis

Arthritis is another disease with an inflammatory component. A recent study indicated that rheumatoid arthritis patients who adopted a Mediterranean diet achieved a reduction in inflammatory activity, an increase in physical function, and improved vitality after following the diet for only three months. There is evidence that oxidation is a factor in the development of rheumatoid arthritis, and some theorize that the antioxidant properties of the diet are responsible for improving the condition. The rich supply of omega-3 fatty acids in the diet is also likely responsible, since these fatty acids have been shown to reduce arthritic symptoms.

Type 2 Diabetes

In type 1 diabetes, for some inborn reason, the body does not produce insulin, which is necessary for the body to be able to use sugar properly. Type 2 diabetes, on the other hand, is acquired; either the body stops producing enough insulin or the cells start ignoring the insulin. It's believed that in most patients, the clinical expression of type 2 diabetes could be prevented by dietary and lifestyle changes. Nearly nine out of ten people with newly diagnosed type 2 diabetes are overweight. Studies have shown that a Mediterranean-type diet can reduce aspects of type 2 diabetes, such as insulin resistance. Since diabetes is associated with a fourfold risk of atherosclerosis, it is of significance that following a Mediterranean diet has also been shown to have a protective role against it for diabetics.

Hypertension

Hypertension has long been recognized as a major risk factor for several common cardiovascular diseases. The World Health Organization reports that three million people will die annually as a result of hypertension. There is evidence to support that the adoption of the Mediterranean diet could help reduce high blood pressure levels. For example, a recent study showed that adherence to the Mediterranean diet as a whole is associated with lower blood pressure, as is olive oil intake in particular. Another study showed that following the diet was associated with a 26 percent lower risk of being hypertensive.

Since **being overweight and obesity are strongly linked to high blood pressure,** losing weight and maintaining weight on the Mediterranean diet can help. I had one overweight patient who came in complaining of headaches, and it turned out he was hypertensive. I was going to start him on blood pressure medications, but he didn't want the expense or hassle, nor did he like that the medications can interfere with sexual function in men, cause allergic reactions, and produce a host of other side effects such as fatigue, abdominal pain, and diarrhea. Instead, he promised me he'd lose weight. I explained my diet and wrote out some recipes on my prescription pad. He went on it, and two months later he had lost twenty pounds. His blood pressure was now normal, and he didn't need any drugs. He was in his mid-thirties, and his father had died of a stroke at a young age, so in many ways this was an extremely successful intervention and lifestyle change.

Metabolic Syndrome

The metabolic syndrome consists of a constellation of factors that increase the risk of cardiovascular disease and type 2 diabetes. The syndrome, also called *insulin resistance syndrome*, consists of three or more of the following characteristics:

- Resistance to the effects of insulin
- High triglyceride levels
- Low HDL ("good") cholesterol
- High blood pressure
- High blood sugar (blood glucose)
- Accumulation of fat around the abdomen

Being overweight is also an important factor, since most of the conditions above are exacerbated if not caused by excess weight.

Many scientists believe that insulin resistance is one of the major factors that either allows or causes the other components of the metabolic syndrome to develop. Insulin resistance, which can lead to type 2 diabetes, does not have symptoms, but a blood test in your doctor's office following a food challenge can diagnose it.

All of the above problems work together to increase the risk of coronary artery disease and kidney disease. It is estimated that one-fourth of the people in the United States may have the metabolic syndrome, and many of them have no idea they have it. If it can be caught in time, the progression to diabetes and heart disease could be halted.

The metabolic syndrome is so strongly associated with diet, weight, and physical activity that lifestyle modification is usually considered front-line therapy, and drug intervention secondary. For example, in one two-year study, patients who went on a Mediterranean-style diet reduced their number of syndrome factors by half—and this finding held true even after being adjusted for weight loss, since the participants also dropped pounds following the Mediterranean program. In another study, the coronary risk associated with the metabolic syndrome fell 35 percent when they adopted a Mediterranean diet. As with the majority of health benefits gained from the Mediterranean diet, the protective effects were found when the diet was taken as a whole, not from the individual components.

Life Span

Certainly the most striking and significant finding about the Mediterranean diet is that it appears to reduce death from *all causes* when compared to other diets. In study after study, the Mediterranean diet is positively associated with longevity. Moreover, it appears that the more you stick to the Mediterranean plan and the longer you follow it, the more you benefit from it. Here is a sampling of the studies that demonstrated increased longevity on the Mediterranean diet:

- A very large study of twenty-two thousand people, published not long ago in the *New England Journal of Medicine*, concluded that greater adherence to the traditional Mediterranean diet is associated with a 25 percent reduction in overall mortality.
- The effects of the Mediterranean diet can even improve health and life span later in life. In one large study of older men (seventy to ninety years old) who'd stayed on the diet for ten years, adherence to a Mediterranean diet and healthful lifestyle was associated with a more than 50 percent lower rate of death from all causes.

THE HEALTH BENEFITS OF LOSING WEIGHT: *There's More to It Than You Think!*

Obesity accounts for around three hundred thousand deaths every year in the United States and will soon overtake smoking as the primary preventable cause of death if current trends continue. Merely being overweight has significant health hazards as well. Given that two-thirds of our population is either overweight or obese, this essentially portends a health crisis. Recent reports have shown that obesity may cut life span by up to twenty years. For overweight people, life span is estimated to be reduced by around three years; for obese people, it's around seven years on average. For grossly obese people (with a BMI over 45), life span may be reduced by as much as twenty years.

It's distressing to me that so much disease and heartbreak for families could be prevented with the aid of diet and lifestyle adjustments. You frequently hear people say things like "Uncle Joe died of a heart attack," or "Aunt Millie died of a stroke," or "My co-worker died of colon cancer." Shockingly, the fact is that being overweight likely contributed or even was fully responsible for their illness. To give one example, in 2003 a ten-year study of nine hundred thousand people reported in the *New England Journal of Medicine* suggested that current patterns of overweight and obesity in the United States account for 14 percent of all deaths from cancer in men and 20 percent of those in women. People who are overweight also have more heart attacks, tend to have them earlier (around four years earlier for the overweight and eight years for the obese) compared with normal-weight patients, and are more likely to have a repeat heart attack. The effects of obesity on cardiovascular health can even begin in childhood, increasing the risk of developing coronary artery disease as an adult.

In addition to the better-known consequences of elevated weight, such as heart disease, diabetes, cancer, and stroke, being overweight can adversely affect virtually every organ and system in the body: the endocrine system and hormones; the digestive system; the lungs, bones, joints, and muscles; the skin; the brain, spinal cord, and other parts of the nervous system; the immune system; and even the eyes. It can cause health problems ranging from hair loss and sexual dysfunction to slow wound healing and birth defects. Indeed, an astonishing array of health problems can be caused by being overweight or obese. (For a more complete description of the damage being overweight does to your body, please refer to Appendix A.)

How Even Modest Weight Loss Can Greatly Improve Your Health

Irrespective of how you drop the pounds, losing a small amount of weight can reduce the presence of illnesses as well as health-risk factors such as high blood pressure and high cholesterol. For example, even modest weight loss can lower cholesterol counts dramatically, thus reducing the risk of coronary disease. Shedding just 5 to 10 percent of your total body weight in a one-year period is often all it takes—even ten pounds can make a big difference in your health. It is clear that with weight reduction we can decrease hypertension and directly and indirectly decrease the incidence of heart disease. Most people can lower their blood pressure by losing 10 to 20 percent of their total body weight.

Here is an example of how a small amount of weight loss can improve your health if you're overweight or obese:

- Type 2 diabetes can be reduced or eradicated with weight loss of only eight to ten pounds (or around 7 percent of starting weight) along with increased physical activity, even more effectively so than with medication.

- Modest weight loss of ten to fifteen pounds may prevent arthritis of the knee from developing and is likely to relieve symptoms and delay disease progression if it already exists.

- Weight loss lowers triglycerides and LDL cholesterol while raising HDL cholesterol; weight loss of 5 to 10 percent can reduce total blood cholesterol.

- Weight loss of as little as 5 percent can reduce high blood sugar, which predisposes one to type 2 diabetes.

- Weight loss of about 10 percent of initial weight is effective in improving menstrual regularity, ovulation, hormonal profiles, and pregnancy rates.

As a practicing physician who actively engages my patients in losing weight to treat themselves, I see wonderful success stories all the time. People are often surprised when I write out recipes onto my prescription pad instead of expensive drug protocols. They're intrigued, even amused. But the best part is when I hear from them a month or two down the road, and they've lost weight and their symptoms are gone.

Take Anthony. He was an obese patient of mine who complained of fatigue, and people were telling him he snored a lot. Sleep apnea and snoring are common among obese people, and both conditions contribute to daytime fatigue, so I wasn't surprised. Anthony also had liver function abnormality as a result of excess fat in his liver (which has now become the leading cause of hepatitis in the United States). I told him he needed to lose weight, so I described my diet and wrote him some recipes on my prescription pad. He came back six weeks later having lost eighteen pounds. He repeated the liver function test, and all of the parameters were improved. Because of Anthony's lifestyle change, he didn't need a CAT scan, a sonogram, or a liver biopsy. His symptoms had all resolved, including his snoring and daytime sleepiness and fatigue.

Another patient I'm going to tell you about only because he did not succeed at managing his eating habits. Lou is five feet five inches tall and weighs 209 pounds; his family and I affectionately refer to him as "Louie Close to the Floor." There is nothing that Lou wouldn't do for me except stop eating. Born in Sicily, he immigrated to the United States twenty-five years ago. In the last fifteen years he gained forty pounds. Accompanied by his wife, he came to see me complaining of increasing shortness of breath and a cough, which were worse at night and after eating. His symptoms had progressed to the point that he could no longer climb the stairs to go to his bedroom. After examining him, I told him that he had asthma and I could make his symptoms go away with medications, but if he lost weight he could minimize the number and quantity of medications that he would have to take or possibly eliminate them altogether. His response to me was, "Doctor, you may find it difficult to believe, but I don't eat anything—I'm starving myself." His wife was sitting next to him and saying nothing, but she was rolling her eyes in disbelief. I gave him my diet and a number of medications and asked that he return to see me in one month.

A month later when I saw him and asked how his diet was going, his response was that he was hungry all the time and he could no longer stay on his diet. He said he "would rather die of shortness of breath than of starvation." Again his wife was staring at the ceiling, rolling her eyes. I got him on the scale, and he now weighed 218—an increase of nine pounds!

The story of Louie Close to the Floor is not that uncommon. People will deny what they're eating and the symptoms that it gives rise to so that they can keep eating the way they always have. To this day my patient is still unable to lose weight and remains on a multitude of medications to control his symptoms, accepting their side effects and costs so that he can continue to eat. If he were to lose even ten pounds from his starting weight, he would improve his glucose tolerance and other symptoms of the metabolic syndrome, breathe easier, and most likely would need fewer medications, and maybe none.

Body Mass Index: Weighing the Risks

Most people believe that the condition of being overweight is easy to recognize. Many also feel that a few extra pounds are normal and safe and that they do not have much to concern themselves with until they begin to tip the scale toward obesity. However, there is actually a fairly narrow range that scientists have determined is a healthy weight for you, and where you rank on this scale may surprise you. The scale they use—the body mass index, or BMI—factors in both height (body surface area) and weight and attempts to predict the amount of body fat you carry. Since excess weight is the cause of more illness than virtually any other medical condition, knowing your BMI is a crucial step toward monitoring your overall health.

Calculating your BMI rather than simply stepping on a scale is a new way of thinking—but because this is how the scientific studies measure weight, this is the only way you can compare yourself to their research. It should become as essential a number to you as your blood pressure and cholesterol levels.

HOW TO CALCULATE YOUR BMI

Multiply your weight (in pounds)_______ × 704 = __________

Take the above amount and divide by your height (in inches) squared, and that's your BMI.

Or

(Your weight in pounds × 704) ÷ (Your height in inches)^2 = Your BMI

If you prefer the metric system, the formula looks like this:

Your weight in kilograms ÷ (Your height in meters)^2 = Your BMI

For example, if Melissa is five foot two and weighs 160 pounds, this is how you would calculate her BMI: $(160 \times 704) \div (62)^2 = 29.3$

So Melissa would be considered overweight, and not far from being obese.

HOW TO USE YOUR BMI CALCULATION

In 1998, the National Institutes of Health (the federal government's principal health research institution) defined five classes of weight based on BMI: underweight, acceptable weight, overweight, obesity, and morbid obesity. The last of these means that a person's weight is so high that it affects his or her normal activities and/or is directly responsible for causing medical conditions or diseases. The breakdown is shown below:

These definitions, widely used by the federal government and now by the broader medical and scientific communities, are based on evidence that **health risks increase more steeply in individuals with a BMI greater than 25, and they continue to increase as BMI increases.**

The predictions, however, are not absolutes. First, the scale may *overestimate* body fat in athletes and others who have a muscular build, indicating that they are overweight when they are not; and second, the scale may *underestimate* body fat in older persons and others who have lost muscle mass, possibly indicating they have a healthy BMI when in fact they are at risk of poor health.

Weight Class	BMI
Underweight	Less than 18.5
Acceptable weight	18.5–24.9
Overweight	25.0–29.9
Obese	30.0–39.9
Extreme or morbid obesity	40.0 and above

Note that this scale is for adults only. Calculating your child's fat ratio is very important, since being overweight isn't healthy for children, either, and it can lead to them being overweight as adults as well. However, this is best done by your child's doctor.

CALCULATING YOUR IDEAL WEIGHT

If you want to calculate a goal weight for yourself, you can do the BMI calculation backward. Let's say that five-foot-eleven Henry decides that he wants to go on a diet and reach the bare minimum in the low-risk category, a BMI of 24.9. He would use the following calculation:

$$\textbf{Desired BMI} \times (\textbf{Height in inches})^2 \div \textbf{704} = \textbf{Desired weight}$$

So for Henry, that would be $24.9 \times (71)^2 \div 704 = 178.3$ pounds, his goal weight.

There is considerable debate these days about what your true goal weight should be, however. For example, a very recent study published in the *Journal of the American Medical Association* concluded that people's goal BMI should be 25, and that having a BMI of 25 to 30 (currently considered overweight) does not increase mortality. They found that a BMI of 18.5 to 24.9 had increased mortality in comparison to a BMI of 25 to 30 (underweight and obesity were still associated with significant increases in mortality). In spite of this analysis, it is my opinion that the NIH guidelines still hold, since it may be that better medications and management are what's keeping overweight people in better shape, and that these data do not reflect a true health advantage to having a BMI in the overweight range. In addition, this article flies in the face of a multitude of other investigations, upon which the federal guidelines were based. Basically, the jury is still out.

Watching Your Waistline

It is not just your weight but also your shape that affects your health. If you have excess fat, where on your body are you carrying it? If you carry excess fat in the abdominal area (giving you an apple-like shape), you are at higher risk for certain conditions such as heart disease, high blood pressure, and diabetes. In contrast, if you are more pear-shaped, carrying excess weight on your hips, thighs, and buttocks, your risk is not as high (though weight loss may be a tougher challenge, since fat in these locations is broken down by the body much more slowly than abdominal fat). There is evidence that these shape correlations hold true even for children: essentially, children with chubby tummies have more heart disease risk factors that may affect them in later life than their pear-shaped peers.

Scientists used to measure your waist-to-hip ratio, but now the prevailing thought is that waist size itself is more important than the ratio. Generally speaking, the above health risks begin to climb when your waist is greater than thirty-five inches if you are a woman and forty inches if you are a man.

2

How to Lose Weight

In this chapter I am going to teach you how to lose weight at a rapid rate. Consider this the beginning of your new life eating healthily, feeling great, and never feeling hungry or unfulfilled. It's the simplest plan in the world, and if you follow it, you *will* lose weight, as I have seen with my patients over and over again. My Two-Week Weight Loss Stage is designed to get you to lose five to ten pounds if you follow it closely. If, however, your goal weight requires you to lose more than this, then you may stay on the plan until you've reached your goal; my patients have lost twenty, thirty, forty pounds and up this way.

Many of my overweight patients initially approached me with the same question: "Dr. Acquista, do you have something for me to lose weight?" They were looking for a miracle cure. One patient was in my office with her husband and asked if she could do acupuncture to decrease her appetite. Her husband affectionately replied, "Sweetheart, you don't need acupuncture pins on your ears, you need spears." Most patients, however, were looking for a magic bullet in the form of a pill. Though they are often willing to take on the expense and potentially harmful side effects of diet pills, I never prescribe them. I don't believe in short-term solutions.

Instead, I put my patients on the Mediterranean Prescription and teach them how to change their diet and exercise habits.

On the next couple of pages I will describe the basic principles of the diet, and after that I provide a two-week menu as an example of what you can eat. This is only a suggestion, though; you have complete freedom to choose a menu you like that follows my rules. Feel free to mix up the order and combinations, and to season to your taste. Feel free to use recipes not included in this book. **You can eat out** if you like as well, as long as you know what ingredients are going into the preparation and the food follows the guidelines.

Because I love to cook and found that my patients were more inspired if they had great-tasting recipes to follow, I have always written out some recipes of mine for my patients on my prescription pad. I now also bring these to you in my recipe section. My goal with the Mediterranean Prescription is to provide easy-to-make, delicious recipes with simple ingredients, as I firmly believe that a weight-reducing meal plan needs to be realistic if it is to have any chance of becoming a part of your life. There is no training, counting, or timing to my plan, just a straightforward menu and recipes. The basic principles are as down-to-earth as my recipes.

I apologize to those of you who are vegan or vegetarian, as this diet will probably not be a good fit for you. I would suggest trying to substitute with tofu, but we didn't eat tofu in Sicily, so I don't have any recipes for it. The Maintenance Stage, however, is largely plant-based, so it would be possible to follow most of my recommendations there with a few substitutions.

DR. ACQUISTA'S TWO-WEEK WEIGHT LOSS STAGE

Here is the daily plan:

Breakfast

- 1 cup of coffee or tea—no dairy or sugar
- 1 slice of multigrain or whole-wheat toast, no topping like butter or jelly
- And/or, hard-boiled egg whites or egg-white omelet, as much as you like

Lunch

- As much fish or seafood of any kind as you like (not battered or fried); eat until you feel very full. Sauces should be based on vegetables, olive oil, and/or vinegar, not cream or butter or margarine. *Or* up to half a chicken (not battered or fried, no skin). For sauces, the same rules apply as with fish.
- As much salad and vegetables as you want, but no potatoes or other starchy vegetables.
- Salad dressing should be olive oil and vinegar, or olive oil and lemon (no bottled salad dressings).
- No bread.

Dinner

- Follow the same plan as for lunch, eating as much fish as you want, or up to half a chicken, plus salad and vegetables.

Snacks

- The goal of this plan is that you will eat enough for lunch and dinner so that you won't be hungry for snacks.
- If you do get hungry, you can have more of what you ate at lunch or dinner.
- Drink as much water, sparkling water, or diet soda as you want, but no juices.

Dessert

- After you've lost the weight you desire, fruits, nuts, and other healthy desserts will be reintroduced into your diet.

Alcohol

- After you've lost the weight you desire, alcohol can be reintroduced into your diet.

Physical Activity

- Exercise daily if possible.

The Basic Principles

1. **Eat a big breakfast if you like.** While the original plan from Dr. Saita included only a hot beverage and a piece of toast, the

one thing my patients have complained about over the years is that they'd like to eat more for breakfast. Because of this, I've allowed for the toast to be supplemented with as many egg-white omelets or hard-boiled egg whites as you like. Just remember—no juices during this time period, as they have too much sugar.

2. **Have a big lunch and dinner.** The idea is to fill up on seafood (any kind, such as fish, shrimp, mussels, or lobster), chicken, and vegetables at lunch and dinner, so that you are not hungry for snacks or dessert. Make twice the amount of food you might normally make. To fill up on fish, you may need to eat almost a pound instead of the third of a pound you may be accustomed to. The same goes for vegetables. Save what you don't finish, and if you do get hungry in between meals, you may snack on what you have left over.

3. **Use olive oil generously.** You'll notice that for a diet book, my recipes use a lot of olive oil. That is because olive oil is good for you and because oil is what makes food taste good, and the only way to make this a permanent way of eating is to use recipes you think are genuinely delicious. Even though the Mediterranean Prescription may technically be considered "high-fat," with 30 to 35 percent of calories from fat, if you minimize red meat and other high-saturated-fat products as I suggest, you are replacing bad fat with fat that's good for your body and your weight.

4. **What is not in any of these recipes: bread (except for breakfast), rice, pasta, or red meat.** Cheese is only used in minimal amounts as a treat. You can add these back eventually, but not during the initial weight loss stage.

5. **Engage in daily physical activity**. Exercise is an important aspect of the plan, and should, as I'm sure you know, be incorporated as a way of life continuing on after the initial phase. It doesn't have to be marathon training—just get moving. At a minimum, walk one mile per day. Instead of sitting down in front of the television after dinner, go for a walk. Ten city blocks away and ten blocks back is about one mile and would not take much time out of your day. Exercise will counter the

tendency of your metabolic rate (the rate at which you burn calories) to slow down as an effect of losing weight. If you can manage a more rigorous exercise routine or are already following one, by all means go for it.

6. **Remember that you have to be very strict in the Two-Week Weight Loss Stage.** This means no extra snacking off the plan! Call it a "tough love" plan if you wish, but it's the only way that really works. I find that when people are overweight, they're addicted to food. It's a useful analogy, because it must be treated in the same way as any other kind of chemical addiction, which is cold turkey. For example, if I were to give people the freedom to snack in between meals, they would prepare the listed snack and eat it—and then they'd usually go on to eat more because they'd started the process.

I also find that people don't count everything they put into their bodies as they eat throughout the day, but in fact all of those nibbles add up. A patient and friend, Maria Burgio, kept telling me, "Doctor, I've been following your plan religiously, but I just can't lose the weight." I asked her what she was eating, and she recited my diet plan, just as I'd told it to her. But one morning we were sitting on her picturesque terrace on the island of Sardinia, and she was lamenting once again about not being able to lose weight. "Maria," I said, "you say you're following the diet, but what about the sugar you just put in your coffee?"

"Well, it was only two teaspoons," she said.

"And what about the cream?"

"I only use a little cream," she replied.

"And I saw you eating cookies earlier."

"Yes, but I don't eat the whole box—I only have three or four!"

Just then her housekeeper appeared at the doorway with a tray carrying a prosciutto sandwich on a croissant. I started laughing.

"Well," she said, "I only have them a couple of times a week. . . ." The great thing is that she did see the error of her ways, and when she really did start following the plan, she lost twenty-five pounds.

So the first phase is designed to rid you of bad habits like those, your oversights, your cravings, and your junk food compulsions. Trust me on this. After you have lost the desired weight, we'll reintroduce snacks, fruits, desserts, cheese, pasta, and so on, but you have to be disciplined initially. Remember your goals of feeling leaner, healthier, younger, more attractive, and better about how your clothes fit. While it may be difficult for some people at the start, ask any thin person anywhere who has lost weight to get there, and he or she will most assuredly agree with the following: "Nothing tastes better than thin!"

How Exercise Helps You Lose Weight for Good

I'm going to go into exercise a little bit now, since one of the greatest predictors of long-term weight loss is whether you exercise or not. As I've said previously, you don't have to be an exercise fanatic—consistency and enjoyment are the most important factors, as opposed to what kind of activity you're doing. Exercise will help you lose weight faster (in a healthy way), help counteract a slowdown in how fast you burn calories, and prevent weight regain. Moderate exercise also helps reduce appetite. It's possible to lose weight and maintain it without exercise, but exercise has many advantages in getting you to where you want to be.

Exercise is especially important if you are losing weight at a fast rate, which my diet enables you to do. It is estimated that when people lose more than two pounds of weight a week, 30 to 40 percent of the weight lost will be muscle. Low-calorie and fast-acting diets result in more muscle loss than fat loss so that the most useful tissue is preserved for times of starvation (fat produces nine calories of energy per gram compared with only four calories per gram produced by your muscle tissue). This is a disaster if you're trying to keep weight off in the long term, because muscle is five times more metabolically active than fat tissue. Muscle determines the overall metabolic rate of the body, so if muscle is lost, the metabolic rate will drop. This means that when the dieter returns to a normal pattern of eating, the lower metabolic rate will result in rapid weight gain. The aim of an exercise program is to lose fat without losing muscle and without reducing metabolic rate.

Aerobic exercise—exercise that gets your heart rate up—is especially useful in this regard: it metabolizes calories, builds muscle, and raises the metabolic rate. Heart rate should be raised to a comfortable level (120 to 130 beats per minute) for twenty to thirty minutes at least three times per week. Aerobic exercise will also raise the metabolic rate for up to twenty-four hours after you have finished training. This helps to burn up extra calories and prevents the metabolic rate from declining. Additionally, resistance training such as weight lifting may not help you lose pounds, but it will increase muscle tissue, which is a good thing (see more on this below).

I hesitate to recommend specific amounts of exercise, because anything is better than nothing. However, studies do suggest that there may be a minimum amount of exercise that will make a difference during weight loss. One recent eighteen-month study of more than two hundred men and women showed that about forty-five to sixty minutes a day was required, though this level wasn't as effective in the first six months as it was by month eighteen. Generally, the more vigorous the activity, the less time you need to do it. As an example, one mile of walking equals one mile of running, but it takes less time to run that distance. My personal preference is to exercise more vigorously to save time, but either way will help you lose weight and gain health benefits. There is also some evidence suggesting that anywhere from thirty to sixty minutes of exercise of *any* intensity at all has about the same effect on weight loss (though longer duration and more intensity do seem to better contribute to weight *maintenance*). In any case, you should be able to reduce the amount of exercise after you've lost the weight you want, if you desire.

An important point to remember while you're losing weight and exercising is that lean muscle tissue weighs a lot more than body fat of equal volume. Thus, if you remain sedentary during your weight loss, the pounds coming off are deceptive. You will be losing weight from heavy muscle first, so people think they've lost more fat than they actually have. Conversely, if you start exercising regularly, your actual body weight may stay the same, or even rise, during the early stages of your new lifestyle regime because you're losing fat and gaining muscle. For this reason I would avoid scales at first. A tape measure or how your clothes fit would be a better marker of your progress, and it will no doubt be affirming that you are getting healthier and leaner.

If you've been sedentary for a long time or have any health problems or health risks, speak to your doctor about finding the best exercise program for you.

THE TWO-WEEK WEIGHT LOSS MEAL PLAN

One busy working couple who tried the Two-Week Weight Loss stage told me that they had fun spending a Saturday afternoon shopping and cooking for their week ahead. They then wrapped up the dishes and stored them in the refrigerator and freezer so that their meals mainly required nothing but heating. While I recommend preparing the meals fresh to maximize flavor, and though the meals don't take much time to prepare, this is one way to cope if you are extremely limited for time. Keep in mind that you can mix and match recipes (there's no special order) and that you can eat out or order in as long as you stick to the principles of the plan.

Breakfast, Days 1–14

- 1 cup of coffee or tea—no dairy or sugar
- 1 slice of multigrain or whole-wheat toast—no butter or jelly
- May also have hard-boiled egg whites or egg-white omelete (can use Egg-Beaters, a vitamin- and mineral-supplemented commercial egg-white mixture), as much as you like. Two suggestions:
  - Scramble 4–5 egg whites (or about ½ to ¾ cup Egg Beaters) to make an omelet, cooking with 1 teaspoon olive oil, adding any vegetables you like except for potatoes or other starchy vegetables; season to taste; no cheese.
  - Boil 4–5 eggs, remove the yolks, and eat the whites with a dash of salt and pepper.

LUNCH AND DINNER

Day	Lunch	Page	Dinner	Page
1	Broiled Chicken	205	Salmon with Orange and Lemon	185
	Swiss Chard with Tomatoes	152	Boiled String Beans and Onion	155
2	Tomato and Tuna Salad	140	Broiled Chicken with Garlic and Lime	206
	Lentil Soup	145	Chickpea Salad	140

Day	Lunch	Page	Dinner	Page
3	Salmon Tartare	186	Halibut N.S.E.W.	181
	Watercress, Onion, and Endive Salad	141	Sautéed Baby Spinach	156
4	Broiled or Grilled Shrimp with Thyme	189	Scrod Filet with Onions and Tomatoes	182
	Sautéed Broccoli	157	Sautéed Cauliflower	158
5	Broiled Chicken with Orange and Lime	206	Broiled Swordfish	191
	Lentil Soup	145	Broiled Asparagus	153
6	Sweet and Sour Tuna	183	Broiled Chicken with Balsamic Vinegar	207
	Boiled Escarole	161	Baked Eggplant	151
7	Baked Tilefish	193	Broiled Chicken with Lemon	207
	Minestrone Soup	145	Baked Zucchini with Eggplant and Tomatoes	152
8	Tuna with Cannellini Beans	184	Sweet and Sour Red Snapper	194
	Broiled Zucchini	160	Sautéed Broccoli Rabe	157
9	Baked Halibut	181	Chicken Cacciatore	203
	Tomato and Onion Salad	140	Shrimp Cocktail	188
10	Calamari Marinara Fra Diavolo	198	Boiled Lobster	190
	Arugula Salad with Onion	142	Sautéed Brussels Sprouts	160
11	Chicken with Garlic and Vegetables	204	Broiled Red Snapper	195
	Broiled Portobello Mushrooms	154	Boiled Broccoli Rabe	158
12	Warm Scallop Salad	139	Chicken Scarpariello	204
	Boiled Zucchini	159	Broiled Eggplant	151
13	Baked Chicken with Tomatoes	205	Striped Bass Oreganato	195
	Minestrone Soup	145	Boiled Romaine	161
14	Scrod with Tomatoes and Capers	183	Whiting in Brodo	196
	Baked Onions	155	Sautéed Swiss Chard	153

GROCERY SHOPPING TIPS

- **I suggest stocking up on anything that will last two weeks**—spices, oils, many vegetables, and nonperishables—at the beginning of the first week, getting enough for the entire stage.
- See my section on **stocking your pantry and refrigerator** in Chapter 3. It will give you guidance on what to keep on hand so you'll have all of the ingredients to whip up many of these recipes.
- **Chicken and fish** should be bought as you go, since they must be cooked or frozen in the first couple of days—though I strongly recommend eating fresh chicken and fish over frozen. Frozen just does not have the wonderful flavor and texture that fresh does (this is especially true for fish).
- **To best store fish,** remove it from the store wrapping and rinse. Dry it well with a paper towel. Then get a new paper towel and wrap the fish in it. Over that, wrap it tightly in a clingy plastic wrap such as Saran Wrap. Then put it in the fridge. This advice was given to me by a sushi chef, and it really helps keep the fish fresh.
- If you keep **citrus** refrigerated, it should last for two weeks longer. But try to buy it more frequently because the longer you store it, the more flavor it loses.
- **Tomatoes** last longer *un*refrigerated, and taste better that way, too!
- While at the supermarket, avoid aisles that may tempt you off the plan!

A Short Note on Transitioning

After you've reached your goal weight, or would like to move on from the two-week plan, it is time to shift to the next phase of the Mediterranean Prescription. Some will want to dive right into the Maintenance Stage, which generally ensures a healthy, steady weight as well as improved health. Others, however, may prefer to transition more slowly into what may be a foreign way of eating.

Switching from an all-you-can-eat-type diet to a plan that's somewhat portion-controlled can also be a booby trap for some people. If you feel you will struggle to give up unlimited portion sizes, then transitioning might be a good idea for you. A patient of mine went on an Atkins-type low-carb, all-you-can-eat diet for fourteen months and lost an impressive forty pounds. However, the diet was so limiting that he eventually couldn't stay on it anymore, and after he went off it, he gained *forty-two* pounds. He told me, "I felt like the diet taught me bad eating habits. I could eat as much as I wanted, and after I did that for a while, I got pretty used to it. So I went off it, and in no time, I weighed even more than when I started." Many studies show that his experience is not uncommon—you may well have encountered it yourself.

During the transition stage, you can add in elements of the Mediterranean Prescription's Maintenance Stage, including food items you may well have been craving, like fruit, bread, and pasta, so that by the end it will feel like a natural way of eating to you. Some might elect to add these foods back into their diets at a measured pace—perhaps one category added every week over a couple of months. That is up to you. As you reintroduce these foods back into your diet, you should find yourself naturally reducing your portions of chicken and fish.

You may also continue to lose weight while transitioning, albeit at a slower rate of around one to two pounds per week, depending on your starting weight, gender, age, and physical activity. The main goal is that at the end of the transition stage, you will be on the full Mediterranean Prescription and following the healthiest diet we know to keep you in robust health and reduce the risk of disease.

3

Slim and Healthy: A Prescription for Life

The Mediterranean diet is one of the easiest diets to adopt and maintain on a long-term basis because it does not require radical restriction of fat or carbohydrates. In fact, I *encourage* a plentiful amount of fat—especially in the form of olive oil—because it's good for you and it tastes good. I also *encourage* carbohydrates—whole-grain breads, cereals, and pastas—because of the many health benefits they bestow. Nor is the Mediterranean Prescription a radical alteration in eating habits; rather, it is just a shift toward more healthful choices. Studies routinely show that it is more palatable and easier to adhere to (undoubtedly the two are related!) than other diets.

In this section I'll advise you on how to eat once you have lost the weight you want to lose—my suggestions will both keep you healthy and prevent weight regain. I've included helpful tips and day-to-day coping strategies to get the most out of the Mediterranean Prescription.

DR. ACQUISTA'S MAINTENANCE STAGE

THE MAINTENANCE STAGE IS DETAILED IN CHAPTER 1, WHERE I HAVE BROken it down into twelve guiding principles. It makes up the bulk of the book because it is the most important, as it provides a road map for healthful eating once the diet is over—for the rest of your life. Be sure to review the pyramid on page 18, since you are following the Mediterranean Prescription only if you are following the appropriate proportions of food types and lifestyle recommendations.

Eating Throughout the Day

It's probably not news to you, but one thing to keep in mind is that it is important to have breakfast, lunch, and dinner at regular intervals, instead of eating one large meal and having little or nothing at other times of the day. Not eating all day and then eating a lot at dinner and later is a typical obesity pattern. Generally people who aren't hungry in the morning have been eating straight from dinner until bedtime and have consumed way more than they think (or will admit) they did. One of the common traits of obese people is that they consistently underreport how many calories they think they are eating. Many people snack during nighttime TV watching as a matter of habit, instead of out of hunger, and aren't entirely aware of how much food they're ingesting. But of course your body knows, and subsequently you aren't going to be hungry for breakfast or lunch the next day. If you are eating more during the day, you'll feel less hungry at night, and the cycle will be broken.

Another important fact is that not eating all day can be a factor in promoting reduced energy needs. The process of digestion itself uses up calories—it's called the thermic effect of food. If you don't eat for a long period (overnight all the way to the following dinnertime), you trigger the metabolic-rate survival mode, meaning you'll burn calories at a slower pace. In contrast, frequent eating is associated with an increase in the thermic effect of food, resulting in more calories being burned. This is the reason so many diets recommend regular meals and snacks.

Eating regularly throughout the day also keeps you from getting hungry and bingeing. You don't want to get to the point where you feel so famished that you gulp down whatever you can get your hands on, not even giving your stomach a chance to tell your head you're full. Uncontrolled eating like this is a recipe for weight gain.

You don't have to eat the minute you get out of bed, but eat at some point in the morning. Portion out midmorning and/or midafternoon snacks, using the Mediterranean Prescription pyramid as your guide. Ultimately, the most important factor in gaining or losing weight is the total amount of calories you're putting into your body; eating at regular intervals just helps you manage what that amount is.

Exercise

While only three out of ten Americans are physically active on a regular basis, and four out of ten aren't active at all, it appears that the majority of people who are able to maintain weight loss are exercisers. They have made activity a part of their life routine, like brushing their teeth or doing laundry. They also use it to keep their weight in check if they start to gain a few pounds. Exercising a little more than normal in a given week can easily head off a rise on the scale.

See pages 64–71, for my recommendations on how much exercise to aim for.

Beating Weight Gain as You Age

Many adults gain weight slowly over time. There is a significant increase in the prevalence of obesity as adults move from the third decade of life (twenty to twenty-nine years) to the sixth decade (fifty to fifty-nine). It is of note that in general, physical activity decreases during this same period. Even small decreases in calorie intake can help avoid weight gain, especially if accompanied by increased physical activity. For most adults, cutting back 50 to 100 calories per day may prevent this gradual weight gain. Another approach is to burn off an extra 100 calories per day by walking at a moderate pace for sixty minutes or briskly for thirty.

See pages 64–71 for more tips on increasing your level of physical activity to improve your health and help prevent weight gain or regain.

Weight Management

Once you have lost the weight you want to lose, how do you keep from gaining it back, as so often occurs? **Regular maintenance is key** so that the problem doesn't get out of hand again. It's *much* easier to lose three pounds than twenty! How your clothes fit is an effortless gauge as to how you're doing; weighing yourself about once a week or so is an option, too. Losing a few pounds can be as simple as cutting back a little on meals for a couple of days or adding an exercise session or two to your week. If you want to make management easy on yourself, micromanage. If you've overindulged one day, just cut back the next or exercise a little more. This will prevent even a few pounds of weight gain.

If you really have gone off track and the pounds have crept back on, resume the Two-Week Weight Loss Stage.

Making Healthy Choices

You don't always have the option to make perfectly healthy food and beverage choices, but you often have a choice that's health*ier* than the others. Making healthier food choices on a daily basis may seem like a small act, but living your life like that adds up to fewer calories and a much healthier diet.

Here is a list of healthier, lower-calorie substitutes for some less-healthy favorites:

FOOD ITEM	**HEALTHIER CHOICE**
White bread	Whole-grain bread
White rice	Brown rice
Butter	Olive oil, olive oil spray
Eggs	Egg whites, Egg Beaters
Whole milk	Skim milk
Sour cream	Puréed cottage cheese, low-fat sour cream, yogurt
Jelly	Fresh fruit, all-fruit jelly
Cake with frosting	Angel food cake with fresh fruit
Apple pie	Baked apple with fruit juice and cinnamon
Ice cream	Sorbet, frozen fruit, low-cal soft serve

FOOD ITEM	HEALTHIER CHOICE
High-fat cookies	Ginger snaps, vanilla wafers, Fat-Free Fig Newtons, graham crackers; watch out for hydrogenated (trans) fats, including in reduced-fat cookies
High-calorie food additives such as cream-based sauces, cheese, and ketchup	Condiments to add flavor with few calories: mustard, horseradish, lemon or lime juice, salsa, vinegar, all-fruit jelly, herbs; sprinkle a small amount of grated cheese instead of using cheese slices
Sugar	Sugar substitute
Red meat	Lean cuts of red meat, or substitute chicken or fish
High-calorie candy such as candy bars	Licorice, jelly beans, hard candy, sugarless candy or mints, sugarless gum
Potato chips and other snack foods high in saturated or trans fats	Air-popped popcorn, nuts, baked chips, pretzels (preferably whole-wheat), Sun Chips, Zany Corn, Soy Crisps, whole-wheat pita chips, brown rice cakes, and other healthier versions of chips; check the labels for ingredients (especially fats) and calories, and portion it into a bowl so you don't mindlessly overeat
Mashed potatoes with butter	Puréed cooked cauliflower with olive oil, a little half-and-half, salt, and pepper (even your kids won't know the difference)

Additionally, you can often make an unhealthy choice healthier. Here are some examples:

- Remove skin from chicken, especially if the chicken has been fried.
- Cut fat off red meat or poultry, preferably before cooking.
- Press a napkin over a hamburger or pizza puddled with oil to sop up some of the grease.
- Pour skim milk over your cereal instead of higher-fat dairy.
- Dilute juice with sparkling water.

- Go for diet soda instead of the sugar-loaded variety; if you think you don't like the flavor of diet soda, try all the different kinds you can find.
- Ask a waiter for olive oil to dip your bread in if you only see butter on the table.
- If you're used to eating bagels or toast with butter, jelly, and/or cream cheese, eat the whole-grain kind and top it with all-fruit jelly, low-fat cream cheese, or a small amount of another kind of melted low-fat cheese (and skip the butter altogether).
- If you're at a buffet, pile on the most nutritive, low-cal choices, and just take small bites of higher-calorie dishes.
- Get a grilled chicken sandwich instead of a fried chicken sandwich.
- Peel the cheese off a cheeseburger (or better yet, order a veggie burger instead).
- If anything comes in a lower-calorie version, go for that.

Of course, in an ideal world, I'd recommend you keep hamburgers and American-style pizza to a minimum, but if you're going to eat them, eat as healthy a version as you can. It doesn't have to be all or none.

FOOD FOR KIDS

Kids learn to eat from their parents. They are often reluctant to try new foods and sometimes won't accept strongly flavored foods until they are grown (kids have a lot more taste buds than adults). So keep in mind that the vast array of foods available on the Mediterranean Prescription gives you and your kids a lot of choices without trying to get them to eat something they hate. The foods that are available in the home are very important. Instead of buying potato chips, make popcorn as a family treat. Keep plenty of fruits in sight and available. Kids would just as soon have an apple or tangerine as a sugary snack. Pack raisins and dried berries with lunches as dessert for your children.

When I was growing up in Sicily, my extended family all ate together, from the children to the grandparents. There were no separate meals cooked for the kids. That's why I don't have a separate recipe section for kids. I feel my recipes are really family recipes. When there are ingredients your kids won't like, simply leave them out or replace them with something they'll like. That said, here are some ideas that are particularly child-friendly and follow the principles of my Mediterranean Prescription.

MEALS

- **Breakfast cereals made of whole grains, with fresh fruit added in.** Use low-fat or skim milk instead of whole milk; they'll still get their calcium, but with much less saturated fat.
- **Slow-cooked oatmeal with raisins, apricots, figs, or dates added in.** Remember, instant oatmeal is highly processed so that it'll cook fast, so some of its health benefits get lost. Avoid instant cereals with added sugar, creamer, and hydrogenated fat.
- **Grilled cheese.** Make it with 2 slices of whole-wheat or multigrain bread. Use cheese low in saturated fat, such as part-skim mozzarella. If your kids are American-cheese snobs, mix the mozzarella in with the American-cheese, and/or buy fat-free or low-fat versions of American cheese. Instead of spreading the bread with butter or margarine, spray it with olive oil spray. It's so delicious using olive oil, your kids will never miss the butter (and you might try it, too).
- **Peanut butter and jelly.** Once again, use whole-grain bread. Choose a peanut butter without trans fats (look for the word *hydrogenated* on the label and avoid it). Instead of jelly loaded with sugar, use all-fruit jam with no added sugar. Or instead of jam altogether, place slices of bananas on the peanut butter.
- **Spaghetti.** There's hardly a family kitchen that doesn't prepare this universal children's favorite regularly. But instead of refined pastas, use whole-wheat or semolina-based pasta. Try it with fresh, homemade sauce with no chemical additives, like Mom's Quick Tomato Sauce later in this

book. If you're going to use prepared sauce, look for brands with added vegetables and little or no sugar added.

- **Pizza.** I'm not talking about the kind that has a thick crust and is loaded with high-fat cheese. See my recipe for healthy, Italian-style pizza on page 178.

Snacks

- **Fruit,** both fresh and dried. Enough said.
- **Vegetables**, cleaned, cut up, and served with low-fat salad dressings, hummus, or peanut butter (sans trans fats).
- **Nuts.** When I was a boy, a handful of nuts was a common snack. It's a great way to get protein and fiber.

HOW TO STOCK YOUR PANTRY AND FRIDGE

An important skill to learn is how to eat and cook the Mediterranean way on a daily basis. To this end, it's imperative that you keep some basics on hand so that your options are Mediterranean-style. It doesn't have to be Mediterranean cuisine per se, but Mediterranean Prescription in spirit.

Keep Stocked in Your Refrigerator

Fruits and vegetables: vegetables such as zucchini, broccoli, broccoli rabe, Swiss chard, cauliflower, brussels sprouts, eggplant, mushrooms, carrots, celery, leeks, bell peppers, escarole, endive, spinach, frozen peas, arugula, romaine lettuce and other salad greens—always have at least two to three vegetables on hand; apples, peaches, oranges, lemons, limes, pears, and other fruits; avocadoes; scallions; olives; pickles; tomato and other vegetable juices

Herbs and spices: fresh herbs (e.g., basil, sage, parsley, oregano, rosemary, thyme, cilantro, mint); ginger

Oils, vinegars, and condiments: soy sauce; jelly (low-sugar with lots of fruit); horseradish; ketchup; lime juice; Dijon mustard; hot sauce

Dairy: grated Parmesan or Pecorino Romano cheese; low-fat milk; eggs

Seafood/Meat: seafood (eat it the same day you buy it if possible); chicken; lean cuts of red meat

Miscellaneous: hummus and other dips for snacking, such as eggplant, olive dip, and tzatziki (a Greek yogurt-cucumber dip); peanut butter (without trans fats); water

Keep Stocked in Your Pantry or Cupboards

Fruits and vegetables: tomatoes and grape tomatoes; onions; dried fruits such as prunes, dates, apricots, and others; potatoes; berries

Grains: bread; spaghetti; whole-wheat flour; brown rice

Legumes: dried lentils; fava beans

Herbs and spices: fresh garlic; sea salt; peppercorns; red pepper flakes; dried oregano; dry mustard; cumin; bay leaves

Oils, vinegars, and condiments: plenty of olive oil; canola oil; sesame oil; balsamic vinegar; red and white wine vinegars; Marsala wine

Canned or jarred goods: canned tuna, sardines, anchovies, and mackerel; canned tomatoes (such as plum, crushed, and diced); tomato sauce; chickpeas; capers; cannellini beans; hot cherry peppers (or milder cherry peppers in vinaigrette); clam juice; vegetable, chicken, and beef stock

Miscellaneous: red and white wine; walnuts, almonds, and other nuts

I keep the above stocked in my kitchen at all times. I buy fresh fish, fruits, and vegetables on a regular basis, but otherwise I have all of the ingredients to whip up a delicious, healthy meal. If fresh produce is too costly, certainly the canned varieties are an option, although not as tasty; just watch out for added ingredients such as sugar and corn syrup (which is mostly sugar).

As you become familiar with the recipes in my book, you'll become more adept at ad-libbing in the kitchen. For example, the Scrod Filet with Onions and Tomatoes can be made with any other kind of fish, or with chicken. You can also cook any fish or chicken with just a little olive oil, salt and pepper, a dash of lemon, and any other seasoning you like. Here are some ideas for throwing a meal together in no time flat.

- The easiest lunch in the world is to open a can of mackerel or tuna, drain the olive oil, add chickpeas from a can, slices of onion and tomato, a little vinegar, salt, and pepper, and you're ready to eat.
- One of the quickest things to prepare among my recipes is the Pasta Alla Crudaiola. The sauce consists of raw garlic, parsley, and olive oil, and instead of fresh tomatoes you can use canned diced tomatoes. The sauce takes about four minutes to prepare, and by the time the pasta is ready it's about fifteen minutes total. While the pasta is cooking, throw some broccoli rabe in another pot and boil. It's incredibly fast, delicious, and healthy.
- Another easy meal is my boiled onions and string beans recipe. I'll add potatoes to it, boil for twenty minutes, pour a little olive oil and dash of salt and pepper on it, and I'm done. It's very filling as a meal in itself.

MAINTENANCE MEAL PLANS

THE ONE-WEEK MEAL PLAN I'VE PROVIDED HERE IS ONLY TO BE TAKEN AS AN example. You don't need to try to follow it day by day. You don't need to measure out the portions I've included here—they are only to give you an *idea* of how much to eat. Choose the fruits you like, the grains you like, the recipes you like, the beverages you like, the desserts you like, and so on, as long as you are following my twelve guiding principles and the daily servings I recommend for each category throughout the book. While eating at least three meals a day is important for your metabolism and to deter hunger attacks, how you divide up what you have for lunch and dinner is not important. With this menu, I merely wanted to illustrate for you what typical days might look like following the Mediterranean Prescription on the Maintenance Stage. Each day totals about 2,100 calories. As you can see, there is room to eat full, delicious meals, as well as to snack and have dessert. You should never feel deprived on the Mediterranean Prescription. (An asterisk means the recipe can be found in Chapter 4.)

DAY 1

BREAKFAST	APPROXIMATE PORTION SIZE
Strawberries	1 cup
Mushroom omelet	2 eggs
Whole-grain bread	1 slice
with olive oil	2 tsp
Cappuccino, low fat	1 cup

LUNCH	
Veal Piccata*	3 oz. veal
Sauteed Broccoli*	1/2 cup
Salad with Mixed Vegetables	1 cup
and Mediterranean Dressing*	1 Tbsp
Plums	1/2 cup

DINNER	APPROXIMATE PORTION SIZE
Broiled Halibut*	3 oz. fish
Spaghetti with Olive Oil and Scallions*	1 cup
Roasted potato wedges	1 cup
with rosemary, drizzled with olive oil	1/2 Tbsp
Sauteed Brussels Sprouts*	1 cup
Fresh tomato	1 tomato
with olive oil	1 Tbsp
and balsamic vinegar, salt, and pepper	

DESSERT	
Orange slices with	1 orange
candied almonds	1 Tbsp

TWO SNACKS	
Yogurt, low fat	3/4 cup
Dates and walnuts	2 Tbsp each

DAY 2

BREAKFAST	APPROXIMATE PORTION SIZE
Mixed fruits	1/2 cup
Whole-grain bread	1 slice
with almond butter	1 Tbsp
Café latte, low fat	1 cup

LUNCH	
Shell pasta with Salmon*	1 1/2 cups
Cucumber slices with tomato and sliced onions	3/4 cup
Whole-grain bread	1 slice
with olive oil	2 tsp
Apple	1 apple

DINNER	APPROXIMATE PORTION SIZE
Broiled Chicken with Garlic and Lime*	4 oz. chicken
Spaghetti with Baked Tomatoes*	1 cup
Spinach salad with	1 cup
Italian dressing	1 Tbsp
Whole-grain bread	1 slice
with olive oil	1 Tbsp

DESSERT	
Peach slices	1/2 cup

TWO SNACKS	
Whole-grain pita bread	1/2 pita
with hummus	1/4 cup
Baby carrots and	8 carrots
grape tomatoes	5 tomatoes

DAY 3

BREAKFAST	APPROXIMATE PORTION SIZE
Grapefruit sections	1/2 cup
Asparagus and Pea Frittata*	1 1/2 cups
Mixed-grain bread	1 slice
with olive oil	1 Tbsp
Espresso	1/2 cup

LUNCH	
Lentil Soup*	1 1/2 cups
Whole-grain bread	1 slice
with olive oil	1 Tbsp
Mixed green salad with	1 cup
almonds and	1 Tbsp
dried cherries	1/2 oz.
with Italian Dressing	1 Tbsp
Bosc pear	1 pear

DINNER	APPROXIMATE PORTION SIZE
Steamed Lobster* (with	4 oz. lobster
olive oil and lemon as	1 Tbsp
dipping sauce)	2 Tbsp
Whole-grain risotto	3/4 cup
Grilled Asparagus*	1 cup
Tomato slices	1 tomato
with Italian dressing	1 Tbsp

DESSERT	
Blueberries	1 cup

TWO SNACKS	
Yogurt, low fat	3/4 cup
Dried apricots and	1/4 cup
almonds	1 oz.

DAY 4

BREAKFAST	APPROXIMATE PORTION SIZE
Orange juice	3/4 cup
Whole-grain cereal with	1 cup
banana slices	1 banana
Skim milk	1 cup
Dark-roast coffee	1 cup

LUNCH	
Chicken Cacciatore*	3 oz. chicken
Grape Tomato Sauce with Spaghetti*	1 cup
Sauteed Baby Spinach*	1/2 cup
Whole-grain bread	1 slice
with olive oil	1 Tbsp
Raspberries (sprinkled with sugar or sugar substitute if you like)	1 cup

DINNER	APPROXIMATE PORTION SIZE
Scrod Filet with Onions and Tomatoes*	4 oz. fish
Broiled Portobello Mushrooms*	1 cup
Romaine Lettuce with Tomatoes and Onions	1 cup
with Italian dressing	1 Tbsp

DESSERT	
Poached Pears in Chianti*	1 pear

TWO SNACKS	
Whole-grain bread	1 slice
with olive tapenade	1/4 cup
Grapes and	1 cup
hazelnuts	1/2 oz.

DAY 5

BREAKFAST	APPROXIMATE PORTION SIZE
Sliced peaches	1/2 cup
Scrambled eggs with	2 eggs
spinach	1/2 cup
Whole-grain bread	1 slice
with olive oil	1 Tbsp
Cappuccino, low fat	1 cup
LUNCH	
Striped Bass Oreganato*	4 oz. fish
Pasta with Peas, Asparagus, and Tomato Sauce*	1 cup
Grilled zucchini and yellow	1 cup
squash with olive oil and garlic	1/2 Tbsp
Whole-grain bread	1 slice
with olive oil	1 Tbsp
Strawberries drizzled with	1 cup
balsamic vinegar	1 tsp

DINNER	APPROXIMATE PORTION SIZE
Broiled Lamb Chops*	4 oz. lamb
Spaghetti with Tomato Sauce and Arugula*	1 cup
Mixed Green Salad with	1 cup
Champagne Dressing*	1 Tbsp
Whole-grain bread	1 slice
with olive oil	1 Tbsp
DESSERT	
Melon slices	1 cup
TWO SNACKS	
Yogurt, low fat	3/4 cup
Raisins and walnuts	2 Tbsp each

DAY 6

BREAKFAST	APPROXIMATE PORTION SIZE
Yogurt, low fat	3/4 cup
Peach slices	1 cup
Whole-grain bread	1 slice
Tea	optional
LUNCH	
Tomato Soup*	1 cup
Cannellini and Green Bean Salad*	1 cup
Whole-grain bread	1 slice
with olive oil	1 Tbsp
Orange slices	1 orange

DINNER	APPROXIMATE PORTION SIZE
Grilled Shrimp with Thyme*	6 oz. shrimp
Spaghetti with Olive Oil and Scallions*	1/2 cup
Grilled Asparagus*	1 cup
Sliced tomatoes and	1 tomato
mozzarella cheese	1 oz.
with olive oil and balsamic dressing	1 Tbsp
Breadsticks	1 large
DESSERT	
Sandro's Mixed Berries*	1 cup
TWO SNACKS	
Pistachios	1/4 cup
Apple slices	1 apple

DAY 7

BREAKFAST	APPROXIMATE PORTION SIZE
Melon slices	1 cup
Poached eggs on	1 egg
tomato slices	1 tomato
Mixed-grain bread	1 slice
with olive oil	1 Tbsp
Cappuccino, low fat	1 cup

LUNCH	
Whiting in Brodo*	4 oz. fish
Whole-grain pasta bowties	1/2 cup
with olive oil and parsley	1 Tbsp
Baked Zucchini with Eggplant	
and Tomatoes*	1 cup
Whole-grain bread	1 slice
with olive oil	1 Tbsp
Grapes	1 cup

DINNER	APPROXIMATE PORTION SIZE
Grilled Swordfish*	3 oz. fish
Roasted potato wedges with	1/2 cup
olive oil and rosemary	1 Tbsp
Tomato and Onion Salad*	1 cup
with Italian dressing	1 Tbsp
Whole-grain bread	1 slice
with olive oil	1 Tbsp

DESSERT	
Red and green grapes	1 cup

TWO SNACKS	
Pecans and dried cherries	1 oz.
Yogurt, low fat	3/4 cup

* = recipe found in Chapter 4

TEN TIPS

1. Don't diet.
2. Satisfy your cravings.
3. Eat decadently.
4. Snack.
5. Get yourself full with healthy, low-calorie food.
6. Make exercise fun.
7. Educate yourself about nutrition.
8. Maintain scrupulously—it's the key to it all.
9. Take advice from people who have the kind of body you want to achieve.
10. Stop with the excuses already.

Life can be hard and stressful, and good food is one of its great pleasures—you should not be depriving yourself of it, and you probably can't make yourself do without food you truly enjoy over the long run. Our desire to feed our hunger is obviously fundamental to our very survival. In the human body, physiologic systems that are vital to our functioning have redundant mechanisms to get the job done, like an airplane that comes equipped with four engines so that if one or more breaks down, there are several backups to keep everyone up in the air. Hunger is one such excruciatingly important essential, so much so that the wiring in our bodies—the hormones, peptides, neurotransmitters, brain structures, fat, protein, and carbohydrate signals and so on—conspires to keep us eating. The interaction of this astonishing array of mechanisms is so incredibly complex that even the top scientists at the best research institutes in the world still know very little about the big picture.

Therefore, since you really should not expect the magic bullet for weight loss anytime soon—even though lots of people like to claim they've got it—your best strategy is to accept that you will have to take charge of your weight yourself. The tips in this section are coping strategies to deal with hunger and to help you keep going with the Mediterranean Prescription. I am including this section in the Maintenance Stage since I recommend these tips after you have achieved your goal weight.

1. Don't Diet

While I encourage you to try the Two-Week Weight Loss Stage if you need to lose weight, that is not a plan to live your life on. You could lose a hundred pounds on it if you stayed on it for months, but if you don't fundamentally change your eating habits, you'll go right back to where you were once you stop following it, as with any diet. That's why the most important part of my book is the Maintenance Stage—it's not the Two-Week plan that will keep you slim for the rest of your life, it's what comes after.

Most people who keep weight off long-term don't feel like they're dieting, because they've incorporated healthy eating habits so thoroughly into their routine that it feels normal and natural. They have found healthy foods that they enjoy, and they make healthy decisions about the food they eat on a daily basis. You can think of the twelve elements of the Mediterranean Prescription as the twelve-step program for eating healthily. Here are a few examples of simple daily choices that add up to a big result:

- Drinking one cup of skim milk in place of whole milk would save 60 calories a day, or six pounds per year.
- Using a sugar substitute in place of 1 tablespoon of sugar would save 48 calories a day, or five pounds per year.
- Eating low-fat potato chips in place of 1 ounce of regular chips would save 80 calories a day, or eight pounds per year.
- Drinking sugar-free lemonade in place of 8 ounces of regular lemonade would save 98 calories a day, or ten pounds per year.

It's key to find healthy snacks, entrées, and desserts that you really enjoy to substitute for unhealthy ones you crave. If you make an effort to find ones that satisfy you, cravings for the other ones will end. Having delicious, low-calorie recipes is an outstanding way to achieve this goal.

2. *Satisfy Your Cravings*

It's okay to satisfy your cravings now and then; just control your portions. Once you've lost the weight you want, controlling how much you eat becomes much easier. For one thing, you fill up faster; for another, ravenous cravings cease, especially if you're eating at regular intervals throughout the day. Often just a bite or two of whatever it is you're craving will do the trick. That's what I do when dessert time comes and there's a decadent dessert on the table—I'll have a couple of bites only, never the whole thing. You can also find low-calorie foods to substitute for the higher-calorie items you're yearning for. Great low-calorie ways to satisfy a sweet tooth are sugar-free gelatin, sugar-free and fat-free pudding, sugar-free hot chocolate, and sugarless candy. Sometimes when you're feeling like eating something, however, it's just boredom. You can often satisfy that craving with herbal tea, sugarless gum, sugarless mints or candy, diet soda, sparkling water, or water with a wedge of lemon.

3. *Eat Decadently*

Don't deprive yourself: enjoy food and eat decadently from time to time. The ideal way to do this is to find delicious recipes that are also healthy, which I have tried to provide in this book. You may also want to splurge occasionally and go off the Mediterranean Prescription. I would suggest doing this only when you are at your goal weight or have some credit in the bank and are a little under your goal weight. If you're at your goal weight, you should compensate the next day by eating less or exercising a little more. Personally, I keep up a regular exercise routine so that I can eat more than I would otherwise be able to without gaining weight. On the other hand, if you're feeling on the heavy side, you haven't earned the right to pig out, and you should stick to the Mediterranean Prescription.

4. *Snack*

Having a nibble a couple of times a day satisfies hunger and cravings and prevents bingeing—but the key is to snack smart. See the recipe section for some great snack ideas. Remember that not eating for a long period can be a factor in reducing your calorie-burning rate. In contrast, frequent eating is associated with an increase in the thermic effect of food, resulting in more calories being burned. This is the reason so many diets recommend regular meals and snacks.

5. *Get Yourself Full with Healthy, Low-Calorie Food*

To maintain ideal weight, many people recommend not eating to the point of being stuffed. This is great advice, if you can follow it. If you're like some people, though, and live for that button-busting feeling after a meal, do not despair. The secret is to get yourself full with healthy, low-calorie food.

People tend to eat the same amount of bulk, no matter what the calories. They'll fill their plate with the same amount of food. So if, instead of having calorie-dense foods on your plate, you fill up with foods that have a lot of water, air, and fiber, like fruits and vegetables, you'll naturally end up eating a lot fewer calories. You may not realize how similarly satisfied you'll feel afterward.

Here are some filling recommendations:

- Soup is a great start to lunch or dinner if it's a low-calorie version. Avoid soups that are cream-based or have cheese, beef, or added sugar. If you're eating store-bought soup, be sure to check the label, as there are many high-calorie soups out there. If you really want to conserve calories, have a cup of bouillon, which has about 5 calories per serving.

- Eat a salad before or with lunch or dinner. Add as many vegetables as you can. Even a simple salad of lettuce, tomatoes, and oil and vinegar will contribute healthy nutrients and help you feel full.
- Add as many vegetables as you can to entrées and as side dishes.
- Drink lots of water or other sugar-free beverages.
- For dessert, try filling, low-calorie treats such as fruit, nuts, low-fat yogurt, sugar-free gelatin, sugar-free and fat-free pudding, low-calorie soft-serve ice cream or frozen yogurt, or sugar-free ice pops.

6. *Make Exercise Fun*

A female friend of mine recently described to me the interesting dynamic in her aerobics class. She said that it seemed that the heavier women sweated and huffed and puffed through the entire workout, pushing themselves through to the very end, while the slim women took a more relaxed approach, stopping for a bit and resting, or even taking a water break, and then resuming with the rest of the class when they were ready; some even left early. This didn't surprise me at all. I suspect that the heavier women are new to the class and, further, that they won't become regulars. They're pushing themselves to exhaustion and not having any fun, so they'll never be able to convince themselves to show up for the class again and again.

People think exercise has to be a sweat-pouring, backbreaking routine, but that's not necessary to stay fit. Walking is a great way to get active. Start with as much aerobic exercise as you feel comfortable doing, and add more when that gets too easy. Alternatively, you may want to begin with resistance training—slow, repetitive exercise, often with weights—since it's easier. Exercise increases the production of testosterone, which in turn raises mood, energy, stamina, and libido in both men and women. The fitter you get, the more you may want to up the ante in terms of how much you exercise—by jogging instead of walking, say—but you'll be doing so because you're feeling great about your changing body and more energetic from your improvement in fitness.

Some additional suggestions:

- Don't get discouraged when you first start an exercise routine. It can take months for your efforts to really show on your body, even if you're exercising vigorously. This is the hardest time for many people, and it's also when many give up because they feel their efforts are futile. But trust me—if you persevere, it *will* pay off.

- Find an activity you enjoy; it's the only way you'll stick with it.
- Take different kinds of classes at your gym to keep things interesting and fun. Many now offer a diverse selection, such as boot camp, boxing, kick-boxing, stationary bike classes, belly dancing, African dance, and so on.
- Listen to music you love or an audiobook on a Walkman or iPod while exercising if you feel bored with the routine of exercise. It makes exercise infinitely variable even if it's the same old treadmill in the basement. Gyms with TVs also help take the edge off boredom.
- Sometimes you might feel really fatigued and too tired to exercise. At those times, remind yourself that it gets better about ten minutes after you've started. You sort of "wake up," end up enjoying the workout, and leave feeling great.

7. *Educate Yourself About Nutrition*

You've already taken a big step toward living a healthy life by reading this book and educating yourself on how to eat healthily. The more you read and know, the better the choices you'll be able to make on a daily basis. Since nutrition recommendations are always changing, it's important to keep up. My favorite publication is the *Nutrition Action Healthletter*, published by the Center for Science in the Public Interest, a not-for-profit nutrition advocacy organization that takes no advertisements. It's an inexpensive, easy-to-read, bimonthly newsletter that debunks common food misconceptions, keeps you up to date on new nutritional health findings, and fills you in on the sometimes shocking contents and calorie counts of popular restaurant, fast-food, and store-bought foods. Check out their Web site at www.cspinet.org/nah.

8. *Maintain Scrupulously—It's the Key to It All*

Maintenance really is the key to it all. It can be a difficult thing to lose twenty or more pounds. You have to watch what you eat and follow a strict exercise regimen, and do all this while your energy level is down and you're not feeling that great about yourself. It's not that hard to lose one or two pounds, though. Have soup, vegetables, and salad for dinner a night or two, have a good, intensive workout at the gym, and you're probably there. So once you've achieved your weight-loss goal, monitor yourself. Some people do this by regular weigh-ins, while some simply gauge their weight by how their clothes, rings, or watches fit. Personally, I like to keep my weight a few pounds under my upper limit (the weight over which I would feel uncomfortable) so that I can indulge from time to time and not feel overweight.

9. Take Advice from People Who Have the Kind of Body You Want to Achieve

I know losing weight can be hard. Around 60 percent of Americans are now considered overweight, and the number is growing, even among children. It can be so difficult, in fact, that even the professionals can't always conquer the problem: I cannot count the number of diet professionals, personal trainers, and even famous obesity doctors I have known who are overweight. I'm not saying they don't know what they're talking about. Individually, they probably know a great deal about healthy eating, proper posture during a squat, and various diet pills, respectively, but if they are overweight, they have probably not figured out how you *can* achieve your ideal weight, either. Just as important is not sticking to your old beliefs about weight loss if they haven't worked for you. It's important to be realistic and let these notions go if they have not enabled you to achieve lasting success. Seek out the advice of people who both have a knowledge of healthy nutrition and are successful in their own lives with weight management.

10. Stop with the Excuses Already

People put barriers in front of themselves that prevent them from getting serious about weight loss. They feel depressed, frustrated, and helpless. Weight loss comes to feel like a ragingly messy house: it feels so overwhelming to take care of the problem that it continually gets put aside for another day. People come up with reasons for their inaction: they're overweight because of genetics and there's nothing they can do, they're overweight because they have low self-esteem and they need to work it out in therapy before a diet is ever going to work, they're overweight because it is their destiny to eat food as their emotional crutch, they're overweight because they're too busy to put a plan into place, they're overweight because they have to eat out a lot.

Well, I've got news for you: every time you put something into your mouth, you are making a *conscious* choice, regardless of whether you're at a fancy restaurant or eating leftovers from the fridge. If those choices are high-calorie, you're going to stay the weight you are. On the other hand, if those choices have fewer calories than what you're eating now, even if nothing else changes, you will slowly lose weight. Losing pounds and staying at your ideal weight are simply a matter of everyday choices, choosing something healthier over a food that's not so healthy. Genetics certainly play a part and may make things harder for you, but saying it's your destiny is defeatist. The calories-in/calories-out equation is ultimately about physics, uniformly unforgiving for all of us, such that if you're putting in less than you're burning up, you will—you must—lose weight. Unless you have physical limitations, exercise is your choice, too. Have you ever seen an obese long-distance runner?

Waiting for good self-esteem is a backward approach. If you live a life you're proud of, your self-esteem will grow. For better or for worse, having a healthy, fit body is intimately tied to how we feel about ourselves, and sometimes to how others feel about us. As a twenty-eight-year-old female patient who lost thirty-five pounds explained to me: "I'd always felt lousy about my weight. I felt invisible to men and felt chronically self-conscious about my body. One day I just decided I was sick of my weight and that it was coming off once and for all, and I started exercising regularly and reading up on nutrition. Once I started losing weight, men started flirting with me more, and it felt great. Even women seemed friendlier to me. After I lost the weight I started feeling better about myself, and for me I don't think it could've happened the other way around." My ultimate goal is to get you healthy on the Mediterranean Prescription, but if looking great and feeling good about yourself are consequences of that, so much the better!

A lot has been said about another common excuse for not losing weight: seemingly uncontrollable overeating due to emotional upset. This is probably the most complex issue to deal with, because it can go back even to childhood. However, there are coping mechanisms that can be mastered to overcome it. Instead of dealing with problems head-on, people turn to food because it makes them feel better, if only for the short term. To conquer this urge, first identify what emotions trigger you to overeat—be able to identify when you're not really hungry but are just feeling sad or angry or what have you. Then find an effective strategy for coping that doesn't involve food, such as relaxation techniques, going for a walk or run or other exercise, writing down your feelings in a journal, talking to friends, making yourself wait twenty minutes to eat after you feel the urge to binge, going shopping, or reading something interesting. Recognize that you'll feel better with this approach than if you were to give in to the craving, which doesn't actually solve anything and will only add to your feeling bad about yourself.

In addition, sometimes facing and attacking problems in a concerted effort can deter a sense of hopelessness and turning to comfort in food. If one of the problems that is distressing you is being overweight, then reading this book and taking action are excellent steps. Some of the emotional pitfalls you experience now are likely tied up in your weight issues, including health issues brought on by being overweight, so losing weight could break this vicious cycle.

HOW TO EAT OUT

SOMETIMES PEOPLE GIVE UP GOING OUT TO EAT WHILE THEY'RE DIETING, which I think is unnecessary. When you are on the Two-Week Weight Loss Stage of the diet, as long as you follow the principles of the plan, you can eat out. If you're concerned a chicken or fish dish will be cooked in saturated fat, simply ask the waiter. Avoid cream sauces, and if that's all they have on the menu, ask for substitute sauces similar to my recipes (e.g., a simple marinara sauce). Once you're on the Maintenance Stage, follow the guidelines as best you can while dining out. Making healthy choices on a day-to-day basis is your goal. This should leave you the room to indulge in foods off the plan once in a while, guilt-free.

It's true that the only way you can be sure you know what's going into your food is if you prepare it yourself, and sometimes dieters want rigorous control over that to ensure weight loss. That is your decision. My goal, however, is not to teach you how to eat on a diet but how to eat in real life so that you can break the vicious cycle of dieting and weight gain. I recommend that you enjoy the pleasure of eating out in a restaurant, and allow yourself a quick on-the-run meal at a fast-food restaurant if you need to. But don't use eating out as an excuse to throw all of your newfound healthy eating habits to the wind. Use the following tips to help you make healthy, or at least healthier, choices. And if you do splurge and have a big meal out with all the fixings, just remember to cut back the next day to compensate for the flood of calories.

A GUIDE TO CHOOSING HEALTHY MEALS AWAY FROM HOME

- **High-fat foods** may be described as fried, basted, braised, au gratin, crispy, scalloped, pan-fried, stewed, or stuffed.
- **Lower-fat choices** are often described as steamed, baked, broiled, roasted, sautéed, stir-fried, grilled, or poached.
- **Avoid high-saturated-fat meats** such as steak, hamburger, lamb, and fatty pork.
- **If you eat pork,** choose loin or cutlet cuts; if you eat a pork chop, don't eat the fat around the edge.
- **Avoid dishes with lots of cheese, sour cream, and mayonnaise.**
- **Avoid creamy sauces**, such as Alfredo sauce. Sauces made with cream are high in saturated fat as well as calories. Instead, choose a tomato-, vinegar-, or olive-oil-based sauce.
- **Start with a low-cal appetizer such as soup or salad.** Starting to fill up will help you eat less of your higher-calorie entrée. Ask for dressing (preferably olive-oil-based) on the side so you can monitor the portion.
- **Don't empty the bread basket.** Decline it if you are in the Two-Week Weight Loss Stage so you won't be tempted. If you're at risk of mindlessly eating roll after roll, send the basket away after you've chosen a piece. Ask for olive oil to dip your bread into if only butter is on the table. Choose a whole-grain piece if you have the option.
- **Eat a handful of nuts, a piece of fruit, or another small, low-cal snack before you head out to dinner** so you don't overeat once you get there; this will especially help curb your hunger for the bread basket or hors d'oeuvres. Same for cocktail hour or a party: have a snack before so that you won't be ravenous and eat everything they put in front of you, since the choices are usually junk.

- **Order dishes with lots of vegetables.**
- **Try new low-cal items**; expand your palate. For example, try new fish varieties, new vegetables, and new methods of preparation.
- **Eat slowly**. Give your stomach a chance to tell your brain you're filling up.
- **Drink lots of water.**
- **Split meals** if the restaurant you're at typically serves very large portions. There may be a plate-sharing charge, but it will still be less than if you'd ordered two entrées.
- **Choose a salad, soup, or appetizer, or a combination of these as your meal** rather than a large entrée. You're sure to save calories and may save money as well.
- **Split one dessert between two or more people.** You'll often find that just a bite or two does the trick to quench that after-meal sweet tooth—try it!
- **Try sticking to restaurants that offer good, healthy choices**, since once you're there, you're a captive of their menu.
- **Take time to look at the menu** and pick those items that are consistent with the Mediterranean Prescription.
- **Go to restaurants serving Mediterranean-style food**, such as southern Italian, Greek, Spanish, and Middle Eastern.
- **When eating Italian**, eat a modest amount of pasta (stick to the Mediterranean Prescription guidelines) and avoid dishes covered in cheese.
- **Asian cuisine**, while obviously not Mediterranean, can be very healthy. Ask for brown rice instead of white rice. Go for fish, chicken, or vegetarian entrées, and avoid anything fried—this includes tempura dishes—and/or that comes in a sugary sauce.

- **Eat for your ♥.** In some popular restaurant chains you will see a little heart by the menu items. Although these may not be all Mediterranean choices, they are choices that meet the American Heart Association guidelines. Picking these items may help you take the guesswork out of menu choices.
- Even if dishes low in saturated fat and calories aren't on the menu, you may still be able to get a healthy meal, because many restaurants will prepare foods to order if you ask.

SUBSTITUTIONS WHEN EATING OUT

Instead of	Try
Croissants	Whole-grain bread or whole-wheat pita bread
Cream-based soups	Broth- or tomato-based soups with lots of vegetables
Quiche and salad	Soup and salad
Buffalo chicken wings	Peel-and-eat shrimp
Steak	Seared tuna
Hamburger	Broiled steak (lean cut)
Fried chicken sandwich	Blackened chicken sandwich
Chicken-fried steak	Veggie burger with a whole-wheat bun
French fries or potatoes with gravy	Baked potato, brown rice, or cooked greens made without salt pork or lard
Pasta Alfredo	Pasta with marinara sauce or garlic and olive oil
Creamy coleslaw	Coleslaw made with vinegar (without mayonnaise), tossed salad with olive-oil-based dressing, or sautéed vegetables
Hot-fudge sundae or ice cream	Sherbet, sorbet, or frozen yogurt
Chocolate cake with frosting	Angel food cake with fresh fruit

Tips for Eating Fast Food

Fast-food franchises today are offering people healthier, more low-fat alternatives than ever before. Chef's salads, grilled chicken sandwiches, and frozen yogurt are just three examples. Use the Mediterranean Prescription as your guideline when ordering. The following are tips to make your experience as healthy as possible.

- First and foremost, select a fast-food restaurant that offers healthy alternatives to the usual high-saturated-fat formula.
- Avoid hamburgers, as they have too much saturated fat and the buns are usually made of highly refined grains and unhealthy fats.
- If you're planning to get a meal special with a sandwich, fries, and drink, pick the kids' meal to help keep your portions in check.
- If you have a burger, think twice about topping it with cheese, special sauce (usually mayonnaise-based), and bacon—they add fat and calories. Pickles, onions, lettuce, tomato, and mustard add flavor without the fat. I only order a hamburger if it's grilled, not fried on a griddle. If the hamburger's thick, I'll cut it in two and only eat half.
- Some chains now offer a veggie burger, which is a good choice for you—and ask them for a whole-grain bun.
- Many franchises now offer salads. Select a restaurant where you have this option. But beware of salads loaded with calories, such as ones filled with cheese, croutons, ham, bacon, and/or fried chicken and covered in a creamy or Ceasar dressing—these can amount to more calories than one of their sandwiches. Pick off most of the offending items (it's okay to keep a taste of whatever you like) and choose a vinaigrette dressing.
- Opt for the salad bar if it's available (but watch out for high-fat dressings and ingredients).
- A baked potato can be a healthy option, but have it with low-fat yogurt instead of butter, sour cream, or cheese.
- Fish at most fast-food restaurants should be avoided since it's usually deep-fried.

- French fries are an obvious no-no since they're cooked in saturated or trans fat, not to mention the sugar-laden ketchup you'd no doubt drag them through.
- Have water, coffee, tea, or diet soda instead of regular soda.
- Steer clear of chicken nuggets or fried chicken, since they're breaded and fried in saturated or trans fat.
- If you're at a pizza restaurant, order a side salad to eat before your slices. It'll add nutrients and help fill you up on healthy food. Removing some of the cheese will help cut down on calories as well.

SUBSTITUTIONS AT FAST-FOOD RESTAURANTS

Instead of	**Try**
Danish or doughnut	Whole-grain bagel
Pancakes	Eggs
Jumbo cheeseburgers	Grilled chicken, roasted turkey, or even a smaller hamburger with lettuce, tomato, pickles, and onion but without the cheese
Fried chicken	Grilled chicken
Ground-beef tacos or burritos	Chicken tacos or burritos; choose whole-wheat tortillas if they're an option
Fried chicken pieces	Chicken fajitas on pita
French fries	Baked potato with vegetable and/or yogurt topping, or just salt and pepper
Potato chips	Pretzels, air-popped popcorn, or baked snacks
Milkshake	Juice, low-fat or fat-free milk, a diet soft drink or frozen yogurt

4

Dr. Acquista's Family Recipes

THE FOLLOWING RECIPES ARE TO BE USED IN CONJUNCTION WITH THE Mediterranean Prescription. If you're trying to lose weight, follow my guidelines in Chapter 2. If you're on the Maintenance Stage and would like to start eating Mediterranean-style, structure your meals around the pyramid proportions found on page 18, and use the sample menu beginning on page 115 for inspiration. Many of my patients have commented to me that it's the recipes that really make my plan doable, so I encourage you to give them a try! I have made a conscious effort to make them simple, so the majority of them can be prepared in under a half hour.

Most of these recipes have been passed down from generation to generation or were created by my mother or other family members, as well as myself, and some have come from family friends. I am most indebted to my mother, Sara, who contributed so many of the recipes, and who has devoted her entire life to family and cooking. I can fondly remember calling her one day to check in on her and asking, "What are you doing, Mom?"

"I just finished breakfast," she told me.

"So what are you doing now then?" I asked.

"Oh," she said, "I'm getting ready for lunch."

Her life has revolved around food and feeding her loved ones. It was a way of nurturing, as well as a way of relaxing and socializing, which has now become my way of relaxing and socializing. As my father, Salvatore, has gotten older, he now assists my mother in the kitchen. He has become her sous chef, cutting and sautéing and preparing all of the ingredients for my mother to cook with. He now gets involved as a way of being closer to the family.

My brother Dominick has also picked up the family hobby and has contributed several recipes. He is a devoted family man who loves to cook—if you call him on any given night at five o'clock, he's home, cooking for his family. He has made this his utmost priority, which I greatly admire him for. He also looks out for his extended family, following traditions from our Mediterranean first home. To this day he makes wine at home for the family and delivers it to me, my mother and father, and uncles in five-gallon barrels. He'll also bring cases of olives to my family, which he finds in old-world Italian produce stores in Queens, and my mother marinates using her Sicilian recipes.

I am also grateful to my cousin's wife Letizia Acquista for supplying several recipes for the book. She is an extraordinary chef whom I've greatly enjoyed cooking with over the years. She is a great example of how you can eat delicious Mediterranean cuisine while remaining trim: she's very petite and yet cooks as a hobby and has a voracious appetite for the meals she makes, using many of the recipes I have here.

I have also included recipes from celebrity New York City area chefs whom I respect and admire. I eat in their restaurants frequently and enjoy their cuisine so much that I enlisted them to contribute to the book. Some of their recipes are their signature dishes, which I liked so much I asked for their recipes—I always do this when I love a dish I'm eating in a restaurant.

I have included several recipes from the world-renowned restaurant Cipriani New York, where world-famous aristocrats, movie stars, financiers, artists, and writers come to enjoy the delicious Italian cuisine. These recipes will transport you to Italy and simply must be tried. Sandro Fioriti—whose heart is as big as his stomach—is in my opinion one of the best chefs in the United States. He is a superb Italian chef, and I am grateful he has generously donated several recipes. I have also included recipes from Vittorio Assaf, the owner of the chic and trendy Serafina restaurant group in Manhattan, where they serve wonderful, authentic Italian fare.

He is a very close friend who has the same passion for cooking that I do, and he has shared many recipes with me. Joseph (Sparky) Spaccavento, of Piccolo's in Hoboken, New Jersey, has also added a number of recipes. Sparky is a phenomenal chef. His landmark, destination restaurant honors its hometown native, Frank Sinatra. People make special trips from Manhattan to get there, and Wall Streeters place take-out orders from across the river. Sparky comes from Molfetta, a small town on the Adriatic Sea, and so cooks in a very typical southern Italian style, meaning he uses a lot of fish and fries very little. Michael Vernon is the executive chef at Geisha, a very trendy Upper East Side restaurant in Manhattan that fuses the best of Japanese and French cuisines. While not Mediterranean, I have included an Asian-style recipe of Michael's to show how other cuisines can readily fit into the Mediterranean Prescription plan, as long as you follow its principles.

Buon appetito!

CHEF'S TIPS

I COME FROM A FAMILY WITH A LONG TRADITION OF COOKING. TO HELP YOU get started, I'd like to offer you a few tips in the kitchen that I've found will greatly enhance any meal.

- **Try to use the freshest ingredients you can,** preferably in-season. It's okay to use canned or frozen goods if fresh would strain your budget, but try to treat yourself regularly with fresh fruits, vegetables, and fish for their spectacular flavor and texture.
- **Olive oil** comes in a thousand varieties. Look for extra-virgin oil from the first cold-pressing for the healthiest (and best-tasting).
- When you're **sautéing**, always heat the pan first, before you add the olive oil. Once the oil is hot, add whatever it is you're sautéing.
- I always drizzle a little **olive oil** onto almost everything before I serve it—vegetables, pasta, fish, and meat dishes—as a flavor enhancer. For pasta sauces, I retain about 2 tablespoons of the olive oil and pour it over the dishes just before I serve it. Use with discretion until you reach your desired weight.
- For **salt and pepper**, I prefer coarse salt and freshly ground pepper.

- In my recipes I include the amount of **salt** that I find to provide the most flavor. Feel free to season to taste. If you are on a salt-restricted diet, simply reduce or eliminate the salt from the recipe.

- I recommend using fresh **herbs and spices** for my recipes, since they taste the best and contain the most nutrients this way. However, if you wish, you can substitute the dried kind. Approximately 1 teaspoon of a dried herb is equal to 1 tablespoon fresh.

- While many of my simple **vegetable dishes** are boiled, another way to cook them (and to retain more of their nutrients) is to steam them. If you don't have a steamer, you can construct one easily with a large pot and a metal strainer; just put an inch of water in the pot, put the vegetables in the strainer, and put the pot's lid on. If the lid doesn't fit exactly, it will still steam; it will just take a little longer. For my recipes, when I use reserved cooking water to dilute the olive oil, I use the same amount but from the bottom of the steamer. Whichever way you heat up the vegetables, try not to overcook them.

- When sautéing **onions** in olive oil, cover the pan and stir occasionally until they're translucent, always taking care not to brown or burn them. You can add 1 tablespoon water (or wine, if already a part of the recipe) to the pan to help prevent burning.

- I prefer to broil a **whole fish** instead of filets. Filets dry out when you cook them, so it's harder to make them taste good. At a fresh fish market, they should ask you how you want your fish cleaned. Tell them to scale it, remove the fins, leave the head on, and take the innards out. What really makes fish taste good is the crispy skin; it adds an ocean of flavor.

- When preparing the **canned tuna** recipes, light tuna packed in olive oil tastes the best and is good for you, but drain the oil before you use it (then add fresh oil, salt, and pepper). I prefer brands from Italy, such as Genoa, Progresso, and Pastene.

- For **tomatoes**, try to use the vine-ripened kind. They're tremendously better than the regular, paler grocery-store kind. They're a bit more expensive, but they are worth every penny. Don't store them in the refrigerator, because they'll lose flavor and spoil more quickly; keep them in a cool, dry place. Incidentally, if you can get your hands on them, plum tomatoes from Sicily are the best!

- **Refrigerate salad after it's prepared**, then add olive oil and vinegar just before serving. Salad tastes much better chilled.
- **Some of the recipes here may seem a little foreign to you**, but I encourage you to try everything at least once. I cook these recipes all the time for guests, for celebrity chefs, and for my dearest family and friends, with excellent reviews and demands for repeat performances. I hope you will find them as delicious as I do.

ANGELO ACQUISTA, M.D.
NEW YORK, NY 10022
DEA #		LIC#

NAME ______________________ AGE ______
ADDRESS ______________________ DATE ______
RX ILLEGAL IF NOT SAFETY BLUE BACKGROUND

℞

Salads

THIS PRESCRIPTION WILL BE FILLED GENERICALLY
UNLESS PRESCRIBER WRITES "d a w" IN THE BOX BELOW.

Refill ______ times
NR ______ Label ______
Dispense As Written
BCM

Warm Scallop Salad

SERVES 4–6

2 pounds bay scallops
Salt
Black pepper
5 tablespoons olive oil
2 cups cremini or white mushrooms, sliced
1 cup finely chopped and seeded tomatoes
⅓ cup chopped parsley
¼ cup dark balsamic vinegar
2 to 3 bunches arugula, thoroughly washed and dried, large stems trimmed, and coarsely chopped

Preheat oven to 500 degrees. Put the scallops in a baking pan. Sprinkle them with salt and pepper and drizzle 2 tablespoons of the olive oil over them. Bake the scallops until they are opaque and firm to the touch, about 6 to 8 minutes. Meanwhile, heat the remaining oil in a large skillet over medium-high heat. Add the mushrooms and cook until golden, stirring frequently, about 6 to 8 minutes. Add the tomatoes, parsley, and vinegar to the scallops and combine well. Make a bed of arugula and spoon the scallops onto the arugula and arrange the mushrooms around the scallops. Spoon any pan juices over the plate and serve immediately.

Warm Calamari Salad

SERVES 4–6

3 pounds squid, cleaned, body cut into 2-by-3-inch wedges, tentacles separated and cut in half
Juice of 1 lemon
1 tablespoon salt
2 garlic cloves, finely minced
3 tablespoons olive oil
1 teaspoon black pepper
1 tablespoon chopped parsley

Bring 2 quarts of water to a boil and add squid, salt, and half of the lemon juice. Bring to a boil, then reduce heat and simmer for about 20 minutes or until tender. Drain squid well, removing excess water with paper towels. Place squid into a serving bowl. While squid are still hot, add garlic, olive oil, pepper, parsley, and remaining lemon juice. Mix well. Serve warm.

Chickpea Salad

Serves 1–2

1 teaspoon dry mustard
1 tablespoon red wine vinegar
1 garlic clove, finely minced
1 teaspoon cumin
2 tablespoons olive oil
One 15-ounce can chickpeas, drained and rinsed
⅓ cup Kalamata olives, pits removed
3 tablespoons chopped parsley
2 tablespoons capers
2 plum tomatoes, seeds removed, chopped

In a bowl, mix mustard, vinegar, garlic, cumin, and oil. Add chickpeas, olives, parsley, capers, and tomatoes. Mix well.

Tomato and Tuna Salad

Serves 1–2

One to two 6-ounce cans tuna packed in oil
1 large beefsteak tomato, cut into 1-inch wedges
½ medium onion, sliced
½–1 teaspoon salt
1 teaspoon black pepper
2 tablespoons olive oil
1–2 tablespoons red wine vinegar

Drain tuna and mix gently with tomato, onion, salt, pepper, oil, and vinegar.

Tomato and Onion Salad

Serves 1–2

1 to 2 large beefsteak tomatoes, cut into wedges
1 medium onion, sliced
½ teaspoon salt
1 teaspoon black pepper

2 tablespoons olive oil
¼ teaspoon oregano
1 gherkin cucumber, peeled and sliced

Mix all ingredients in bowl and serve.

In the Maintenance Stage you can add feta cheese and Kalamata olives to make a Greek salad.

Watercress, Onion, and Endive Salad

Salads taste better cold. Keep salad in the refrigerator until ready to serve.

Serves 1–2

1 bunch watercress, thoroughly washed and dried, trimmed
½ medium onion, sliced
1 endive, sliced
2 tablespoons olive oil
1 to 2 tablespoons white balsamic vinegar
1 teaspoon salt
1 teaspoon black pepper

Place watercress in bowl and add onion and endive. Cover with plastic wrap and place in refrigerator for ½ hour. Add oil, vinegar, salt, and pepper. Mix and serve cold.

Cannellini and Green Bean Salad

Serves 4–6

½ medium onion, thinly sliced
5 tablespoons sherry vinegar
1 pound green beans, trimmed and cut into 1-inch pieces
1 teaspoon salt
One 15-ounce can cannellini beans, drained and rinsed
3 tablespoons olive oil
1 teaspoon black pepper

Soak onion for 10 minutes in 3 tablespoons of vinegar. Bring 2 quarts of water to a boil. Add string beans and salt. Boil for 4 minutes, until crisp-tender. Immediately place beans in ice water to stop them from cooking. Drain well and dry beans with a paper towel. Drain vinegar-soaked onions and add onions to bowl with string beans. Add cannellini beans. In a separate bowl, mix oil, remaining vinegar, and pepper. Add oil mixture to the beans and mix gently. Serve at room temperature.

Arugula Salad with Onion

Serves 1–2

2 bunches arugula, thoroughly washed and dried, large stems trimmed
½ onion, sliced
3 tablespoons olive oil
1 tablespoon white balsamic or red wine vinegar
½ teaspoon salt
½ teaspoon black pepper

Place arugula and onion in a bowl. Cover with plastic wrap and chill in refrigerator until ready to serve. Prior to serving, add oil, vinegar, salt, and pepper. Toss well. Serve cold.

ANGELO ACQUISTA, M.D.
NEW YORK, NY 10022
DEA # LIC#

NAME ______ AGE ______
ADDRESS ______ DATE ______
RX ILLEGAL IF NOT SAFETY BLUE BACKGROUND

Rx

Soups

THIS PRESCRIPTION WILL BE FILLED GENERICALLY
UNLESS PRESCRIBER WRITES "d a w" IN THE BOX BELOW.

Refill ______ times
NR ______ Label ______ Dispense As Written BCM

Lentil Soup

A very dear friend of mine, Dr. Valavanur Subramanian, a world-renowned cardiac surgeon who popularized minimally invasive open-heart surgery, always requests this dish from my mother.

SERVES 4

One 14-ounce can crushed tomatoes
5 tablespoons olive oil
½ pound dried lentils
1 onion, chopped
2 carrots, chopped
2 celery ribs, chopped
4 stalks Swiss chard, thoroughly washed, trimmed, and cut into 1-inch strips
1 tablespoon salt
1 teaspoon black pepper

Cook the tomatoes in 1 tablespoon oil for 15 minutes and set aside. Rinse lentils under cold running water. Bring 2 quarts of water to a boil in a 6-quart pot, and add all ingredients, including pre-cooked tomatoes, except 2 tablespoons oil. Bring back to a boil, then lower heat and simmer covered 30 to 40 minutes, stirring occasionally, until lentils are tender. Remove from heat and add remaining 2 tablespoons oil.

Minestrone Soup

SERVES 2–4

One 14-ounce can crushed tomatoes
¼ cup olive oil
1 teaspoon salt
2 carrots, cut into ¼-inch cubes
1 medium onion, chopped
½ head broccoli, cut into florets
1 leek, white part only, thoroughly washed, and chopped
2 celery ribs, cut into ¼-inch cubes
1 cup string beans, trimmed and cut into 1-inch pieces
2 cups frozen peas, defrosted (run water over for 1 minute)
1 teaspoon black pepper

In a large pot, cook the tomatoes in 1 tablespoon of olive oil for 15 minutes on low heat. Add 2 quarts of water and bring to a boil and add salt, 1 tablespoon oil, carrots, onion, broccoli, leeks, celery, and string beans. Bring to a boil, then reduce heat and simmer for 20 to 25 minutes, adding peas for the last 5 minutes. Add remaining oil and pepper to individual bowls.

In the Maintenance Stage you can add pasta and serve as a complete meal.

Tomato Soup

The lycopene in tomatoes is one of the most potent antioxidants that is derived from food. Tomatoes, tomato paste, and even ketchup are good sources of concentrated lycopene.

Serves 8

5 tablespoons olive oil
2 onions, chopped
8 garlic cloves, finely minced
One 28-ounce can crushed tomatoes
One 14-ounce can diced tomatoes
1 quart chicken broth
Two 15-ounce cans cannellini beans, drained and rinsed
4 cups 1-inch cubes dry bread
1 teaspoon salt
1 teaspoon black pepper
14 basil leaves, sliced into strips
½ cup grated Parmesan cheese

In a 6- or 8-quart pot, sauté onions and garlic in 2 tablespoons oil for 3 to 4 minutes. Add crushed and diced tomatoes. Bring to a boil. Add chicken broth. Bring to a boil. Add cannellini beans, bread, and salt and pepper. Bring to a boil again, lower heat, and simmer for 5 minutes. Divide soup among bowls and add basil, cheese, and 1 teaspoon of oil per bowl.

Kale and Bean Soup

Serves 4–6

1 pound dry pinto or red kidney beans (or six 15-ounce cans pinto or red kidney beans, drained and rinsed)
4 garlic cloves
4 sage fresh leaves
2 whole cloves
4 to 6 tablespoons olive oil
1 large onion, halved
1 celery stalk
2 tablespoons tomato paste
2 bunches kale, washed, stems removed, roughly chopped
3 medium potatoes, in ¼-inch dice
Salt
Black pepper
8 slices Tuscan bread

If using dry beans, soak the beans overnight in enough water to cover the beans. Drain. Place beans in a 6- to 8-quart pot and add enough water to cover. Add 1 clove garlic, 2 whole sage leaves, and cloves and boil 20 to 30 minutes, until tender. Drain beans, reserving cooking water. Purée half the beans in a blender and add reserved water to the purée, using only enough water to reach your desired consistency. Crush 2 garlic cloves, finely chop 2 sage leaves and half onion, and dice celery. Heat oil in skillet and sauté crushed garlic, chopped sage, onion, and celery for 2 minutes. Add tomato paste and bring to a boil. Reduce heat and cook for 10 minutes. Add tomato mixture to reserved bean purée mixture. Add kale and potatoes and cook for 30 minutes. Add rest of beans and cook 5 minutes more. Season with salt and pepper. Toast bread slices. Cut remaining garlic clove and rub toast slices with cut side of garlic. Place bread at the bottom of bowls and pour the soup on top of the bread.

Escarole and Bean Soup

Serves 4

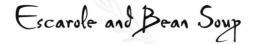

⅓ cup olive oil
4 garlic cloves, sliced
5 anchovy filets
1 teaspoon red pepper flakes
1 pound escarole, washed, trimmed, and chopped about 1 inch long
1 cup cannellini beans, freshly cooked or canned
1 teaspoon salt

Heat the oil and sauté garlic, anchovies, and red pepper flakes until garlic is golden. Add escarole and stir. Add beans, salt, and 3 cups water. Bring to a boil, then reduce heat and simmer 15 minutes, until escarole is tender.

Squash Soup

Serves 2–4

½ cup olive oil
1 medium white onion, chopped
1 pound winter squash, cut into 1-inch cubes
Salt
4 tablespoons grated Parmesan cheese
2 tablespoons minced parsley
2 to 4 slices Tuscan bread
1 clove garlic, halved

Heat oil and sauté onion until soft. Add squash and salt to taste. Cover and cook for 10 minutes, stirring occasionally on medium heat. Add enough water to cover squash and cook for another 30 minutes. Sprinkle with cheese and parsley. Toast bread and rub slices with cut side of garlic to make crostini, and serve with the soup.

ANGELO ACQUISTA, M.D.
NEW YORK, NY 10022
DEA # LIC#

NAME ____________ AGE ______
ADDRESS ____________ DATE ______
RX ILLEGAL IF NOT SAFETY BLUE BACKGROUND

℞

Vegetables

THIS PRESCRIPTION WILL BE FILLED GENERICALLY
UNLESS PRESCRIBER WRITES "d a w" IN THE BOX BELOW.

Refill ______ times

NR ______ Label ______ Dispense As Written BCM

Baked Eggplant

SERVES 4

5 tablespoons olive oil
1 large onion, thinly sliced
3 medium eggplants
6 garlic cloves, halved
4 ounces Romano cheese, cut into slivers ¼ inch thick and 2 inches long (omit to reduce calories)
12 anchovy filets
1 tablespoon salt
1 tablespoon black pepper
One 28-ounce can diced tomatoes

Preheat oven to 375 degrees. Sauté onion, covered, in 1 tablespoon olive oil until translucent, approximately 2 to 3 minutes. Cut eggplants in half vertically and place on flat baking pan, skin down. Make 2 slits in cut side of each eggplant half, taking care not to cut skin. In each slit, tuck half a garlic clove, 1 piece of cheese, and 1 anchovy. Sprinkle stuffed eggplant with salt and pepper and drizzle with remaining oil. Top eggplants with onion and tomatoes. Cover pan with foil and bake for approximately 1 hour, or until eggplant is soft.

Broiled Eggplant

SERVES 1–2

2 medium eggplants, sliced lengthwise ⅓ inch thick
6 tablespoons olive oil
1 garlic clove, finely minced
1 teaspoon salt
1 teaspoon black pepper
1 tablespoon chopped parsley
1 tablespoon white wine vinegar or white balsamic vinegar
½ teaspoon oregano

Preheat broiler. Brush both sides of eggplant slices with 3 tablespoons oil and place on baking pan. Broil 4 to 5 minutes on each side 7 inches from heat source, watching carefully so it doesn't burn. Place in serving dish. Combine remaining oil, garlic, salt, pepper, parsley, vinegar, and oregano and drizzle on top of eggplant. Serve hot.

Baked Zucchini with Eggplant and Tomatoes

Serves 4

2 pounds zucchini, cut into thin strips ½ inch by 2½ inches
1 large onion, thinly sliced
1 medium eggplant, cut into thin strips 1 inch by 3 inches
3 tablespoons olive oil
1 teaspoon salt
1 teaspoon black pepper
One 12-ounce can crushed tomatoes
¼ cup grated Parmesan cheese

Preheat oven to 425 degrees. Place zucchini, onion, and eggplant in large baking dish. Drizzle with oil and mix well. Add salt and pepper and mix again. Top with tomatoes and cheese. Cover with aluminum foil and bake in preheated oven for 40 minutes, or until zucchini is fork tender. Turn oven setting to broil. Remove foil, mix gently, and broil for 3 minutes.

Swiss Chard with Tomatoes

Serves 2–4

1 bunch Swiss chard, thoroughly washed, trimmed, and cut into 1- to 2-inch pieces
1 teaspoon salt
4 garlic cloves, sliced
3 tablespoons olive oil
One 12-ounce can crushed tomatoes
1 teaspoon black pepper

Boil chard in 2 quarts water with salt for 5 minutes. Drain well, reserving 1 cup water, and set aside. Sauté garlic in oil until golden and add drained chard. Sauté for 1 to 2 minutes. Add tomatoes and reserved cooking water and cook, covered, on medium heat for 10 minutes. Season with pepper.

Sautéed Swiss Chard

SERVES 2–4

1 large bunch Swiss chard, washed, stems trimmed
3 tablespoons olive oil
6 garlic cloves, crushed
½ teaspoon salt
½ teaspoon black pepper

Bring 1 quart of water to a boil. Add chard and cook for 4 minutes. Drain well and set aside. In a skillet, sauté garlic in oil until golden. Add chard and sauté for 3 to 4 minutes. Season with salt and pepper and serve hot.

Broiled Asparagus

SERVES 2–3

1 pound asparagus, bottoms trimmed
1 teaspoon salt
1 teaspoon black pepper
2 tablespoons olive oil

Preheat broiler. Place asparagus in a single layer in a broiling pan. Sprinkle with salt and pepper and drizzle with oil, mixing so that asparagus is well coated. Broil for 4 to 5 minutes 7 inches from heat source, watching carefully so as not to burn asparagus. Can also be grilled.

Asparagus and Pea Frittata

Any leftovers make a great lunch the following day.

SERVES 4–6

3 tablespoons olive oil
1 medium onion, chopped
1½ cups frozen peas
1 pound asparagus, bottoms trimmed, cut into 1-inch pieces

1 teaspoon salt
1 teaspoon red pepper flakes
4 egg whites
1 egg
3 tablespoons grated Parmesan or Romano cheese

Sauté onion in oil for 1 to 2 minutes, covered. Add peas and asparagus and cook, covered, until asparagus is fork tender, approximately 6 to 7 minutes. Add salt and red pepper. Mix the egg and cheese together and add to pan, covering the peas and asparagus as evenly as possible. Cook over medium heat for 3 to 4 minutes. When frittata has solidified, place an inverted dish over the pan and turn pan and dish upside down in one motion. Slide the frittata back into the pan and cook the other side for 2 to 3 minutes uncovered. Transfer to a dish for serving.

Broiled Portobello Mushrooms

Serves 2–4

4 portobello mushrooms, cleaned
4 tablespoons olive oil
1 garlic clove, finely minced
1 tablespoon balsamic vinegar
1 teaspoon salt
1 teaspoon black pepper
1 teaspoon chopped parsley
½ teaspoon oregano

Preheat broiler. Toss mushrooms with 1 tablespoon oil. Broil mushrooms, stem side down, for 4 minutes. Turn and broil for 1 minute more. Slice mushrooms into ½-inch slices. Mix remaining oil, garlic, vinegar, salt, pepper, parsley, and oregano, and pour on top.

Baked Onions

Serves 4–6

6 tablespoons olive oil
3 pounds small white onions, peeled
½ cup chicken stock or meat stock
Salt
Black pepper

Preheat oven to 350 degrees. Heat the oil in a large skillet over medium-high heat and sauté the onions until they are lightly browned on all sides, about 10 to 15 minutes. Put the onions in a baking dish just large enough to hold them in one layer and add the oil from the skillet and the stock. Sprinkle with salt and pepper. Bake until the onions are tender, about an hour, turning the onions from time to time and adding a few spoonfuls of stock or water only if they are in danger of burning. When the onions are done, the only liquid remaining in the dish should be the richly flavored oil they cooked in.

Boiled String Beans and Onion

Serves 4

1 pound string beans, trimmed and cut in half
1 tablespoon salt
1 large onion quartered, or 2 medium onions, halved
3 tablespoons olive oil
1 teaspoon black pepper

Bring 2 quarts water to a boil and add string beans, salt, and onion. Cover, reduce heat, and simmer on medium heat 15 minutes. Drain, reserving ½ cup water, and place in a bowl with the reserved water. Drizzle with oil and add pepper. Serve hot.

Sautéed Baby Spinach

Restaurants will normally sauté spinach in oil and butter. It tastes just as good without the butter.

Serves 1–2

3 tablespoons olive oil
4 garlic cloves, sliced or crushed
9 ounces baby spinach, thoroughly washed and slightly wet
½ teaspoon salt

In large frying pan, sauté garlic in oil until golden. Add spinach and cover. When slightly wilted, add salt. Stir the spinach to coat it well with oil. Cook for 4 to 5 minutes total.

Spinach Pie

Leftovers make for a perfect lunch the following day.

Serves 4

½ pound spinach, thoroughly washed, stems trimmed
1 teaspoon salt
4 egg whites
1 egg yolk
2 tablespoons grated Parmesan or Romano cheese
1 teaspoon red pepper flakes
3 tablespoons olive oil
3 garlic cloves, crushed

Boil the spinach in 2 quarts of water with salt for 2 to 3 minutes. Drain spinach well and put in a large bowl. In a separate bowl, beat egg whites with yolk and mix in the cheese. Add half the beaten egg mixture to the spinach. Add red pepper. In a nonstick frying pan sauté garlic in oil until golden. Remove garlic from pan, add the spinach and egg mixture, and cook over medium heat. Add the remainder of the beaten egg mixture to the top of the spinach and let cook, covered, until the spinach and egg mixture solidifies, 3 to 4 minutes. Place an inverted dish over the frying pan and turn pan and dish upside down in one motion. Slide the pie back into the pan and cook the other side for 2 to 3 minutes uncovered. Transfer to a dish for serving.

Sautéed Broccoli

SERVES 2

1 bunch broccoli, thoroughly washed and cut into 4 to 6 pieces, stems trimmed
1 tablespoon salt
4 tablespoons olive oil
6 garlic cloves, sliced

Bring 2 quarts of water to a boil and add broccoli and salt. Cook for 3 minutes. Drain broccoli very well. Heat 3 tablespoons oil in a frying pan and sauté garlic until light golden, approximately 30 seconds. Add broccoli and sauté 2 minutes, stirring to coat broccoli with oil. Place in serving dish and drizzle with remaining oil.

Sautéed Broccoli Rabe

SERVES 1–2

2 tablespoons olive oil
6 garlic cloves, crushed
1 bunch broccoli rabe, washed and trimmed
½ teaspoon red pepper flakes
½ teaspoon salt

Sauté garlic in oil until golden. Add broccoli rabe and red pepper flakes and sauté for 1 minute, stirring constantly. Add ¼ cup water and salt and cook for another 3 minutes.

Boiled Broccoli Rabe

Serves 1–2

1 bunch of broccoli rabe, thoroughly washed and trimmed
1 teaspoon salt
1 tablespoon olive oil

Bring 1 quart of water to a boil and add broccoli rabe and salt. Bring to a boil again and boil for 2 minutes. Drain, reserving ¼ cup water. Mix broccoli rabe, oil, and reserved water and serve hot.

Sautéed Cauliflower

Serves 2–4

1 head cauliflower, thoroughly washed and cut into 3-inch pieces
1 teaspoon salt
5 tablespoons olive oil
4 garlic cloves, chopped roughly

Bring 2 quarts of water to a boil and add cauliflower and salt. Boil 3 to 4 minutes, then drain well. In a frying pan sauté garlic in 3 tablespoons oil until light golden, about 30 seconds. Add cauliflower and sauté 2 to 3 minutes, stirring to coat cauliflower with oil. Before serving, drizzle with an additional 1 to 2 tablespoons olive oil.

Sweet and Sour Cauliflower

Serves 1–2

3 tablespoons olive oil
1 garlic clove, finely minced
½ head cauliflower, cut into florets
1 large tomato, seeded and diced
2½ tablespoons red wine vinegar
1 teaspoon salt

In a large nonstick frying pan, over medium heat, sauté the garlic in oil for 30 seconds. Add the cauliflower, tomato, vinegar, and salt. Cover and cook for 7 minutes or until cauliflower is tender.

Boiled Zucchini

SERVES 4–6

2 pounds zucchini, cut into 1-inch by 3-inch slices
1 tablespoon salt
2 tablespoons olive oil
1 teaspoon black pepper

Bring 2 quarts of water to a boil and add zucchini and salt. Boil for 5 minutes or until fork tender. Drain, reserving ¼ cup water. Add oil, reserved water, and pepper to zucchini.

Oven-Baked Zucchini

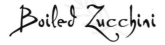

This is a fabulous recipe given to my mother by the sister of Dr. Saita (the doctor who originated my diet plan) when she stayed in our home while Dr. Saita was hospitalized. She had lived with her brother, and because she was elderly and wasn't able to take care of herself while he was away, my family took her in. This is typical in Sicilian culture, where neighbors took each other in when needed. In fact, there were no nursing homes in my town. Family and friends always took care of one another.

SERVES 4–6

6 tablespoons olive oil
2 eggs
1 teaspoon salt
1 teaspoon black pepper
1 cup seasoned bread crumbs
3 medium zucchini, cut into slices ½ inch thick and 4 inches long

Preheat oven to 375 degrees. Put 4 tablespoons oil in a shallow baking pan. In a bowl beat the eggs and add the salt and pepper. In another bowl place the bread crumbs. Dredge the zucchini in the egg mixture, then the bread crumbs. Place the breaded zucchini into the baking dish so that the pieces are not touching one another. Drizzle with remaining oil. Bake for 20 minutes, turn the zucchini, and bake for another 15 minutes, until browned and fork tender.

Broiled Zucchini

Serves 4–6

2 pounds zucchini, cut into pieces ¾ inches thick and 4 inches long
4 tablespoons olive oil
1 teaspoon salt
1 teaspoon black pepper
2 garlic cloves, finely minced
1 tablespoon white balsamic vinegar
1 tablespoon chopped parsley

Preheat broiler. Coat zucchini with 2 tablespoons oil. Place on baking pan and sprinkle with salt and pepper. Broil for about 5 minutes on each side. Mix remaining oil, garlic, vinegar, and parsley and pour over zucchini.

Sautéed Brussels Sprouts

Serves 4–6

2 pounds brussels sprouts, washed and cut in half
1 tablespoon salt
3 tablespoons olive oil
2 garlic cloves, finely chopped
1 teaspoon black pepper

Bring 2 quarts of water to a boil. Add brussels sprouts and salt. Cook until fork tender, about 7 minutes. Drain. In a frying pan over high heat, sauté garlic, brussels sprouts, and pepper in oil for 30 to 40 seconds.

Boiled Romaine

My mother makes this dish whenever someone in our family has stomach problems. You will be surprised at how sweet it tastes. Sicilians think that boiled green vegetables with their broth will cure all stomach ailments.

SERVES 4

2 heads romaine lettuce, thoroughly washed, leaves separated
1 teaspoon salt
2 to 3 tablespoons olive oil
1 teaspoon black pepper

Bring 2 quarts of water to a boil. Add lettuce and salt and cook for 3 to 4 minutes. Drain, reserving ½ cup of water. Mix oil with reserved water and pepper and pour over lettuce.

Boiled Escarole

SERVES 1–2

1 bunch escarole, thoroughly washed and trimmed
1 teaspoon salt
2 tablespoons olive oil
1 teaspoon black pepper

Bring 1 quart of water to a boil and add escarole and salt. Return to a boil and cook for 4 to 5 minutes. Drain escarole, reserving ¼ cup water. Put escarole in a bowl. Add oil to reserved water and mix with escarole. Sprinkle with pepper.

Caponata

Serves 4

4 tablespoons olive oil
1 eggplant, peeled and cut into 1-inch cubes
1 cup chopped fresh tomatoes or canned crushed tomatoes
1 red bell pepper, coarsely chopped
1 green bell pepper, coarsely chopped
1 onion, coarsely chopped
3 garlic cloves, finely minced
20 imported black olives, pitted and chopped
¼ cup capers
¼ cup chopped parsley
2 tablespoons chopped fresh marjoram
2 tablespoons red wine vinegar

In a large nonstick frying pan, over medium-high heat, sauté the eggplant in the oil for 2 minutes. Add the tomatoes, peppers, onion, and garlic. Reduce heat and simmer for 10 minutes, stirring occasionally. Add the olives, capers, parsley, marjoram, and vinegar. Turn the caponata into a large bowl; cover and let sit for at least 2 hours in the refrigerator before serving.

ANGELO ACQUISTA, M.D.
NEW YORK, NY 10022
DEA # LIC#

NAME ______ AGE ______
ADDRESS ______ DATE ______
RX ILLEGAL IF NOT SAFETY BLUE BACKGROUND

℞

Legumes

THIS PRESCRIPTION WILL BE FILLED GENERICALLY
UNLESS PRESCRIBER WRITES "d a w" IN THE BOX BELOW.

Refill ______ times
NR ______ Label ______ Dispense As Written BCM

Many people aren't used to cooking legumes, such as beans, peas, and lentils. I'm including a short cooking tutorial here to help you along, since being unfamiliar with them shouldn't keep you away from such a healthful, filling, delicious part of the Mediterranean Prescription.

Dry bean basics

- Store dry beans in a dry, airtight container at room temperature, and use within one year for best results.
- Remove any bits of foreign matter in the beans.
- Rinse before using to clean and to reduce the gas-producing properties of beans.
- Refrigerate cooked beans and use within four to five days.
- Freeze extra beans in an airtight container and use within six months.

Canned beans—great for convenience!

- Store in a cool, dry place, and use within one year for best results.
- Canned beans are already cooked, so they only need to be reheated.
- Drain the beans and rinse to reduce sodium content and to remove

some of the starchy residue found in the liquid (which helps to reduce problems with intestinal gas).

Soaking legumes

- After sorting and rinsing, use about 3 cups of water for each cup of dried beans or whole peas.
- Quick soak: Bring to a rolling boil for 2 minutes, remove from heat, cover, and let stand for 1 hour; discard water before cooking.
- Microwave soak: Cover and microwave on high for 10 to 15 minutes, then let stand for 1 hour; discard water before cooking.
- Overnight soak: Soak beans overnight and discard water before cooking; beans will keep their shape better and have a more uniform texture than with quicker soaking methods.

Legume	Soak First	Cooking Time
Black beans	Yes	2 hours
Black-eyed peas	Yes	1 hour
Chickpeas	Yes	1½ hours
Kidney beans	Yes	1½ hours
Lentils	No	15–20 minutes
Lima beans (large)	Yes	1½ hours
Navy beans	Yes	1½ hours
Pinto beans	Yes	1½ hours
Soybeans	Yes	2½ hours
Split peas	No	1¼ hours
White beans	Yes	1½ hours

Cooking legumes

- 1 pound of dry beans = about 2 cups of dry beans = 5 cups of cooked beans
- 2 cups of dry lentils = 3 to 3½ cups cooked lentils
- 1 pound canned beans = about 2 cups
- Simmer beans gently, as boiling will cause skins to split.
- Cook beans until just barely tender if they are to be cooked again in a recipe.
- A tablespoon of olive oil added to the cooking water will help to reduce foaming.
- Salt and acids (e.g., lemon juice or tomatoes) will impair the softening process of beans, so add these closer to the end of the cooking time.

Boiled Fava Beans

My favorite bean!

SERVES 4

3 pounds fresh fava beans, shelled, or 2 pounds frozen (in their pods)
6–8 garlic cloves, crushed
1 tablespoon salt
2 tablespoons olive oil

If using frozen beans, run them under warm water for 30 seconds. Bring 2 quarts water to a boil and add beans, garlic, and salt. Cook 20 minutes for fresh beans, 10 minutes for frozen, until tender. Drain, reserving ⅓ cup water. Place in bowl and add reserved water and oil.

If the skins are still tough, you can bite off the tops of the bean and squeeze out the bean from the skin with your front teeth. If the skins are tender, I encourage you to eat the whole bean, as they are a great source of fiber.

Zuppa di White Broad Beans

Serves 4–6

1 pound dry white beans
1 medium white onion, chopped
3 garlic cloves, crushed
Salt
4 whole sage leaves
¾ cup olive oil
2 celery stalks, chopped
2 carrots, chopped
1 medium red onion, chopped
1 sprig rosemary, leaves chopped and stem discarded
3 tablespoons tomato paste
1 bunch Swiss chard, washed, stems trimmed, chopped
1 head cabbage, shredded
Black pepper

Soak the beans overnight in water, enough to cover beans. Drain beans and place in a 6- to 8-quart pot with water to cover beans. Add white onion, garlic, salt, and sage and boil for 30 minutes, until beans are tender. Drain the beans, reserving the cooking water. Purée half the beans in a food processor and add to the reserved water. To a hot skillet add ½ cup oil and sauté celery, carrots, red onion, and rosemary for 5 minutes. Add tomato paste and 1 tablespoon water. Purée this mixture and add to the pureed beans. Add Swiss chard and cabbage and cook 30 minutes. Add the reserved whole beans, remainder of oil, and salt and pepper and cook for 20 more minutes.

Other legume-rich recipes

Chickpea Salad

Cannellini and Green Bean Salad

Lentil Soup

Minestrone Soup

Kale and Bean Soup

Fava Beans with Pasta

Pasta Fagioli

Tuna with Cannellini Beans

ANGELO ACQUISTA, M.D.
NEW YORK, NY 10022
DEA # LIC#

NAME ______ AGE ______
ADDRESS ______ DATE ______
RX ILLEGAL IF NOT SAFETY BLUE BACKGROUND

℞

Pasta and Other Grains

THIS PRESCRIPTION WILL BE FILLED GENERICALLY
UNLESS PRESCRIBER WRITES "d a w" IN THE BOX BELOW.

Refill ______ times
NR ______ Label ______ Dispense As Written BCM

Pasta alla Crudaiola

Serves 2–4

6 garlic cloves, crushed
3 tablespoons chopped flat-leaf parsley
3 tablespoons olive oil
4 tomatoes canned or fresh, peeled, seeded, and coarsely chopped, with their juice
½ pound spaghetti
Salt
½ teaspoon red pepper flakes
¼ cup grated Parmesan

Combine garlic and parsley in a large serving bowl. Heat 2 tablespoons olive oil, add tomatoes, and cook 2 to 3 minutes. Pour tomato mixture over garlic and parsley and stir. Cook the pasta in salted water and drain, reserving 1 cup water. Add reserved water to tomato mixture. Add drained pasta to sauce and mix. Add red pepper flakes and remaining oil to pasta and mix. Sprinkle with cheese.

Spaghetti with Baked Tomatoes

Serves 2–4

4 to 5 beefsteak tomatoes, quartered
4 tablespoons olive oil
3 garlic cloves, finely chopped
1 teaspoon oregano
½ cup grated Romano cheese
1 teaspoon black pepper
1 tablespoon salt
½ pound spaghetti

Preheat oven to 425 degrees. In a baking dish place tomatoes skin side down. Drizzle with 3 tablespoons oil and sprinkle with garlic, oregano, 4 tablespoons cheese, and pepper. Cover the dish with foil and bake approximately 20 minutes. Turn oven to broil. Remove the foil, press tomatoes with a fork to flatten slightly, and broil for 1 to 2 minutes. Cook spaghetti with salt, drain, and toss the tomato sauce with the pasta and drizzle with remainder of oil (1 tablespoon). Sprinkle with reserved cheese.

Spaghetti with Tomato Sauce and Spinach

Serves 4–6

3 tablespoons olive oil
3–4 garlic cloves, crushed
1 teaspoon red pepper flakes
28-ounce can crushed tomatoes
½ pound baby spinach, thoroughly washed and dried, stems removed
1 pound spaghetti
¼ cup grated Parmesan

Sauté garlic and red pepper flakes in oil until garlic is golden. Add tomatoes and cook, covered, 10 minutes. Add spinach and cook 2 minutes. Cook spaghetti and drain. Add the pasta to the sauce and heat for 30 to 45 seconds. Sprinkle with cheese.

Spaghetti with Tomato Sauce and Arugula

Serves 4–6

3 tablespoons olive oil
3–4 garlic cloves, crushed
1 teaspoon red pepper flakes
28-ounce can crushed tomatoes
½ pound arugula, thoroughly washed and drained of all liquid
1 pound spaghetti
¼ cup grated Parmesan

Heat oil and sauté garlic and red pepper flakes until garlic is golden. Add tomatoes and simmer, covered, 10 minutes. Add drained arugula and cook 2 minutes. Cook spaghetti, drain, and add to sauce. Heat for 30 to 45 seconds. Add cheese and stir.

Grape Tomato Sauce with Spaghetti

Serves 4–6

6 tablespoons olive oil
10 garlic cloves, sliced
2 pints small grape tomatoes, halved
Salt
Black pepper
1 teaspoon red pepper flakes
½ cup Tomato Base (see page 227)
1 pound spaghetti
3 tablespoons grated Parmesan cheese

In a large, nonstick skillet, heat 4 tablespoons oil and sauté garlic for 1 minute. Add tomatoes, salt, pepper, and red pepper flakes. Bring to a boil, then reduce heat to medium-low and cook, covered, for 5 minutes, stirring occasionally. Add Tomato Base and cook for 1 minute more. Cook spaghetti, drain, and add to sauce in pan for 30 seconds. Drizzle 2 tablespoons oil over spaghetti and sauce before serving. Sprinkle with cheese.

Spaghetti with Shrimp and Cognac Sauce

Serves 4–6

8 tablespoons olive oil
6 garlic cloves, crushed
1½ pounds medium shrimp, peeled and deveined
Salt
Black pepper
1 teaspoon red pepper flakes
¼ cup cognac
One 28-ounce can crushed tomatoes, or 3 cups Mom's Quick Tomato Sauce (page 227)
¼ cup clam juice
1 pound spaghetti

Heat frying pan over high heat and add 4 tablespoons oil. Sauté garlic until golden and add shrimp, being careful not to overcrowd pan. Sauté shrimp 1 minute on each side. Add salt, pepper, and red pepper flakes. Add cognac and cook for an additional 15 to 30 seconds. Remove shrimp and set aside. In the same pan, heat 2 tablespoons oil and add tomatoes. Bring to a boil, reduce heat, and simmer 10 to 15 minutes. Return shrimp to the pan and simmer for 3 minutes. Add small amounts of clam juice as needed to give a loose consistency. Cook and drain spaghetti. Add to shrimp and sauce and heat through, approximately 30 seconds. Remove from heat and drizzle with remaining oil.

Spaghetti with Red Snapper

My favorite pasta dish.

Serves 4–6

1 pound spaghetti
4 teaspoons salt
7 tablespoons olive oil
1 medium onion, chopped
1 pound skinless red snapper filet, cut into ½-inch cubes
1 teaspoon red pepper flakes
2 tablespoons chopped parsley
½ cup white wine
3 plum tomatoes, seeded and chopped

Boil pasta in water with 3 teaspoons of salt. While the pasta is cooking, in a large pan heat 3 tablespoons oil and sauté onion and fish for 3 minutes over medium heat. Add remaining salt, red pepper flakes, and 1 tablespoon parsley. Add wine and cook for 1 minute, stirring gently. Add tomatoes and cook for 3 minutes. Drain pasta well, then add it to the pan and mix well. Add the remaining 4 tablespoons oil and remaining parsley. The best!

Spaghetti with Olive Oil and Scallions

Serves 2–4

½ pound spaghetti
5 tablespoons olive oil
1 bunch scallions
1 teaspoon salt
1 teaspoon red pepper flakes
2 tablespoons grated Parmesan cheese

Cook pasta. While pasta is cooking, heat 3 tablespoons oil in large skillet and sauté scallions, salt, and red pepper flakes over low-medium heat for 4 to 5 minutes, covered, watching that scallions don't burn (may add 1 to 2 tablespoons water to prevent burning). Drain pasta, reserving 1 cup water. Add pasta and reserved water to skillet with scallion mixture and cook 30 to 40 seconds on high heat. Remove from heat and add remaining oil. Sprinkle with cheese.

Shells with Salmon or Squid

Serves 6

¼ cup olive oil
1 large onion, thinly sliced
1½ pounds salmon filet, cut into 1-inch cubes, or 2 pounds squid, cleaned, body cut into ¼-inch circles and tentacles cut into halves
Salt
Black pepper
1 teaspoon red pepper flakes
1 teaspoon oregano
One 28-ounce can crushed tomatoes, with equal amount of water
1 pound pasta shells
¼ cup grated Parmesan

In a large pan or pot, heat the olive oil and sauté onion until translucent (may add 1 tablespoon water to prevent burning). Add salmon or squid and sauté for an additional 2 minutes. Add salt, pepper, red pepper flakes, and oregano and stir gently. Add the tomatoes and 3 cups water and bring to a boil. Lower heat and simmer for 15 to 20 minutes. In another pot, cook pasta, drain well, and pour sauce over pasta, drizzling with remaining 2 tablespoons oil. Sprinkle with cheese.

Bowtie Pasta with Tuna

This was served to me by the chef on Giuseppe Cipriani's yacht off the coast of Sardinia.

SERVES 4–6

Three 6-ounce cans tuna packed in oil
1 pound farfalle (bowtie) pasta
4 teaspoons salt
8 tablespoons olive oil
1 medium onion, chopped
1 teaspoon red pepper flakes
2 tablespoons chopped parsley
½ cup white wine
3 plum tomatoes, seeded and chopped

Drain tuna and discard oil. Boil pasta in water with 3 teaspoons salt. While pasta is cooking, in a large pan heat 4 tablespoons oil and sauté onion and tuna for 3 minutes over medium heat. Add remaining salt, red pepper flakes, and 1 tablespoon parsley. Add wine and cook for 1 minute, stirring gently. Add tomatoes and cook for 3 minutes. Drain pasta well, then add it to the pan and mix well. Stir in the remaining oil and parsley.

Pasta with Peas and Tomato Sauce

SERVES 4

6 tablespoons olive oil
1 medium onion, chopped
One 10-ounce box frozen peas
One 28-ounce can crushed tomatoes
1 pound ditali, or any short pasta
¼ cup grated Parmesan

Heat 4 tablespoons oil over medium-low heat and sauté onion until translucent. Add peas and sauté 2 to 3 minutes. Add tomatoes and bring to a boil. Reduce heat and simmer, covered, for 20 minutes, stirring occasionally. Cook pasta, drain well, and add to tomato mixture. Heat for 30 seconds. Add remaining 2 tablespoons oil and sprinkle with cheese.

Pasta with Peas, Asparagus, and Tomato Sauce

Serves 4–6

6 tablespoons olive oil
1 medium onion, chopped
One 10-ounce box frozen peas
8 ounces asparagus, bottoms trimmed, cut into 1-inch pieces
One 28-ounce can crushed tomatoes
1 pound ditali, or any short pasta
¼ cup grated Parmesan

Heat 4 tablespoons oil over medium-low heat and sauté onion until translucent, being careful not to burn onion. Add peas and asparagus and sauté for 2 to 3 minutes. Add tomatoes and bring to a boil. Reduce heat and simmer, covered, 20 to 30 minutes, stirring occasionally. Cook pasta, drain, and add to tomato mixture. Heat for 30 seconds. Add remaining oil and sprinkle with cheese.

Fava Beans with Pasta

Serves 4

1 pound shelled fava beans
4 garlic cloves, crushed
1 tablespoon salt
1 pound ditalini or small shells
5 tablespoons olive oil
1 medium onion, diced
1 teaspoon red pepper flakes
¼ cup grated Parmesan cheese or grated ricotta salata

Add beans and garlic to 1 quart boiling water with ½ tablespoon salt and cook approximately 10 minutes if frozen or 20 minutes if fresh, until fork tender. Drain and set aside. Cook pasta with 1/2 tablespoon salt and drain, reserving 1 cup water. In a hot skillet, sauté onion and red pepper flakes in 3 tablespoons oil for approximately 4 minutes. Add fava beans and cook, covered, for 2 minutes. Add drained pasta to beans and reserved pasta water and cook for 1 minute. Add remaining 2 tablespoons oil. Sprinkle cheese on each dish.

Pasta Fagioli

Serves 2–4

2 onions, chopped
¼ pound pancetta or bacon (optional)
1 tablespoon olive oil
1 cup crushed tomatoes
2 cups cannellini beans, pre-soaked
¼ pound ditali pasta
½ teaspoon salt

Sauté onion and pancetta in olive oil until onion is translucent. Stir in tomatoes and 2 cups water. Add beans and cook about 45 minutes, until tender. In a separate pot, cook pasta with salt for 2 minutes less time than package specifies. Drain pasta and add to bean mixture. Cook for another 2 minutes. For a brothier consistency, add ½ cup of the pasta water.

Pizza

I made this pizza frequently for the nurses in the open-heart surgery recovery room at Lenox Hill Hospital while my father was hospitalized. I usually get my dough from pizza restaurants.

Serves 6–8

1½ pints grape or cherry tomatoes, halved and squeezed into bowl
2 garlic cloves
14 basil leaves
1 teaspoon salt
1 teaspoon black pepper
3 tablespoons olive oil
Dough for 1 pizza, at room temperature for 2 hours
5 tablespoons grated Parmesan cheese
¾ pound whole-milk mozzarella (preferably within 2 days of purchase), cut into ½-inch cubes

Preheat oven to 500 degrees. In a large bowl combine tomatoes, their juice, garlic, basil, salt, pepper, and 2½ tablespoons oil. Oil a 12 by 17-inch baking pan with remaining oil. Spread dough in pan. Top dough with tomato mixture, reserving juice, and bake 10 minutes. Remove from oven, top with cheeses, and drizzle with 4 to 5 tablespoons reserved tomato juice. Bake another 4 to 5 minutes, or until bottom is done.

ANGELO ACQUISTA, M.D.
NEW YORK, NY 10022
DEA # LIC#

NAME ________ AGE ________
ADDRESS ________ DATE ________
RX ILLEGAL IF NOT SAFETY BLUE BACKGROUND

Rx

Fish and Other Seafood

THIS PRESCRIPTION WILL BE FILLED GENERICALLY
UNLESS PRESCRIBER WRITES "d a w" IN THE BOX BELOW.

Refill ________ times
NR ________ Label ________ Dispense As Written BCM

Halibut N.S.E.W.

The name of this recipe comes from how my mother described preparing this delicious dish to former New York governor Hugh Carey when he asked her how she made it.

Serves 4–6

1 large onion, thinly sliced
2 Idaho potatoes, thinly sliced (optional)
3 tablespoons olive oil
1½ teaspoons salt
2 pounds halibut steak, 1 inch thick
1 teaspoon black pepper
½ cup white wine

Place the onion in oil with ½ teaspoon salt over very low heat, and add potatoes on top of salted onions. Sauté covered until potatoes are a little tender (about 5 to 7 minutes). Do not lift the lid, but stir the ingredients by holding the handles and moving the pan, as my mother used to say, "north to south and east to west." Do not brown onions. Sprinkle fish with remaining salt and pepper and place on top of potatoes. Pour wine around fish, cover, and bring to a boil. Reduce heat and simmer for 10 to 12 minutes. Do not lift the lid while fish is cooking, but stir by moving the pan "north to south and east to west."

Baked Halibut

This is an easy dish that also works remarkably well with other types of fish, such as scrod, tilefish, and salmon.

Serves 4–6

2 pounds halibut, divided into 4 pieces
4 teaspoons finely chopped ginger
2 teaspoons chopped garlic
½ cup Marsala wine
4 tablespoons soy sauce
Salt
Black pepper
1 tablespoon sesame oil
Juice of 1 lemon

Preheat oven to 400 degrees. Place halibut in baking pan. Mix ginger, garlic, wine, soy sauce, salt and pepper to taste, add sesame oil and pour over fish. Cover dish with foil and bake 10 to 13 minutes. Sprinkle with lemon juice.

Broiled Halibut

This recipe can also be made with red snapper, striped bass, tilefish, black sea bass, or other fish.

Serves 4–6

¼ cup plus 1 tablespoon olive oil
4 halibut steaks, 6 to 8 ounces each
1 tablespoon Dijon mustard
1 tablespoon white wine vinegar
1 large or 2 small tomatoes, peeled, seeded, and chopped
2 tablespoons bread crumbs
2 tablespoons grated Parmesan cheese

Preheat broiler. Grease broiler pan with 1 tablespoon oil and lay fish on pan. Make vinaigrette by mixing mustard and vinegar in a small dish and whisking in ¼ cup oil. Brush fish with vinaigrette. Broil fish for approximately 7 minutes, 4 inches from the heat. Combine remaining vinaigrette with chopped tomatoes and spread over cooked fish. Mix bread crumbs and cheese and sprinkle over the tomatoes. Return fish to broiler for another minute or until tomatoes are warmed through.

Scrod Filet with Onions and Tomatoes

This recipe also works well with a variety of other fish—such as snapper, black and striped bass, and tilapia—as well as chicken.

Serves 4–6

¼ cup olive oil
1 large onion, thinly sliced
2 pounds scrod filet
Salt
Black pepper
1 pint grape tomatoes, cut in half, or 8 ounces diced tomatoes
1 cup white wine

Sauté onion in oil for 5 minutes covered over low heat, being careful not to brown onions (can add 1 tablespoon water or wine to prevent burning). Season scrod with salt and pepper and place over onion. Add tomatoes and wine to pan. Raise heat and bring to a boil. Reduce heat, cover, and simmer for 15 to 20 minutes, depending on thickness of fish. Spoon sauce over the fish.

Scrod with Tomatoes and Capers

SERVES 2–4

1 pound scrod filet
2 tablespoons olive oil
1 teaspoon salt
1 teaspoon black pepper
One 8-ounce can stewed tomatoes, drained and chopped
2 tablespoons capers, chopped
⅓ cup green olives, pitted and chopped
¼ cup white wine
Juice of ½ lemon

Preheat oven to 400 degrees. Lightly coat both sides of fish with 1 tablespoon oil. Place fish in baking dish and season with salt and pepper on both sides. Spoon tomatoes over the scrod and top with capers and olives. Drizzle with wine and remaining oil. Bake uncovered for 15 to 20 minutes. Squeeze lemon juice over fish and serve with lemon wedges along side.

Sweet and Sour Tuna

SERVES 4–6

5 tablespoons olive oil
1 onion, thinly sliced
2 pounds tuna steak, ¾ inch thick
1 tablespoon salt
1 tablespoon black pepper
¼ cup flour for dredging
¼ cup red wine vinegar
8 to 14 Kalamata olives, pitted and halved
1 tablespoon capers, rinsed

Heat 1 tablespoon olive oil in large pan and sauté onion until transparent. Set onion aside. Season tuna with salt and pepper and lightly dredge in flour. Heat 3 tablespoons oil in pan and sauté tuna for 2 minutes. Turn tuna, add onions, vinegar, olives, and capers, and cook for 1 to 2 more minutes. Spoon juice, olives, onions, and capers on top of tuna and drizzle 1 tablespoon oil over top to serve.

Tuna with Cannellini Beans

SERVES 1–2

Two 6-ounce cans tuna packed in olive oil
1/2 red onion, sliced thin
5 tablespoons white or red wine vinegar
One 15.5-ounce can cannellini beans, rinsed and drained
1 teaspoon salt
1 teaspoon black pepper
2 tablespoons olive oil

Drain oil from tuna and discard. Soak onion in 3 tablespoons vinegar for 1 hour. In large bowl gently break up tuna. Add cannellini beans, salt, and pepper. Drain onions and add to tuna and beans, tossing gently. Add oil and remaining vinegar and mix.

Tuna Meatballs

This dish is best as an appetizer.

SERVES 6

1 pound fresh tuna, diced into small pieces
1 egg
6 tablespoons plain bread crumbs
3½ ounces grated pecorino cheese
3 tablespoons minced parsley
2 to 3 tablespoons raisins, soaked in water until plump and dried
2½ ounces pine nuts
Salt
Black pepper
Flour for dredging

8 tablespoons olive oil
2 garlic cloves, finely minced
One 12-ounce can whole peeled tomatoes, drained and diced

Put tuna in a bowl and add the egg, bread crumbs, cheese, parsley, raisins, and pine nuts. Season with salt and pepper. Mix well and shape mixture into balls. Dredge the meatballs in flour, shaking off any excess. Sauté the meatballs in 6 tablespoons oil until cooked through, 1 to 2 minutes. In a saucepan, heat remaining oil and sauté garlic until golden. Add tomatoes and cook 10 minutes. Add the meatballs and cook another 10 minutes.

Tuna Tartare

Serves 4–6

2 pounds very fresh sushi-quality tuna, cut into ¼-inch cubes
1½ tablespoons Dijon mustard
3 tablespoons sesame oil
1 teaspoon salt
1 teaspoon black pepper
3 tablespoons finely chopped ginger
2 tablespoons finely chopped cilantro
½ avocado, peeled and cut into ¼-inch cubes

In a large mixing bowl combine all ingredients and mix gently with your hands. Serve cold.

Salmon with Orange and Lemon

Serves 4–6

Juice of 1 orange
Juice of 1 lemon
1 tablespoon soy sauce
3 tablespoons olive oil
2 pounds salmon filet
Salt
Black pepper

In a large baking dish, combine orange juice, lemon juice, soy sauce, and olive oil. Season salmon on both sides with salt and pepper. Add salmon to juice mixture and marinate in the refrigerator for 45 minutes per side. Preheat broiler. Broil salmon 6 inches from heat source for 10 to 12 minutes. Spoon the cooked juice over salmon and serve immediately.

Salmon Tartare

Serves 2–4

1 pound very fresh sushi-grade salmon, cut into ⅓-inch cubes
½ avocado, peeled and cut into ⅓-inch cubes
1 teaspoon salt
2 tablespoons sesame oil
1 tablespoon finely chopped ginger
1 tablespoon finely chopped cilantro
1 tablespoon Dijon mustard

In large bowl combine all ingredients and gently mix with your hands. Serve cold.

Miso-Marinated Salmon

This recipe is from Michael Vernon, executive chef at Geisha in Manhattan.

Serves 4

1 cup sake
1 cup mirin
½ cup shiro (blond) miso paste
Four 6-ounce salmon filets
2 tablespoons canola oil
16 medium-size shiitake mushrooms, stems removed
2 garlic cloves, roughly chopped
1 small knob ginger, roughly chopped
Salt
Black pepper
8 scallions, trimmed to about 8 inches long

Combine sake and mirin in medium-size pot and boil until reduced by half. Place miso in a bowl and slowly whisk in the sake-mirin mixture. Strain and cool completely. Brush a thin layer of sauce onto salmon filets. Let salmon marinate for at least 4 hours in refrigerator. Heat 2 tablespoons canola oil and sauté mushrooms, bottom (white) side up, 1 to 2 minutes until lightly browned. Add garlic, ginger, and a little water to cover the bottom of pan and simmer until mushrooms are tender. Season with salt and pepper and set aside. Blanch scallions in boiling salted water for 20 to 30 seconds, until tender, and plunge into ice water. Preheat broiler and broil marinated salmon 3 to 4 minutes, until medium rare. Gently heat the mushrooms in a casserole. Warm the sauce in a small casserole. Season scallions with salt, brush with a little canola oil, and broil. On a large plate, make a line of mushrooms. Lay the salmon on the mushrooms and place the scallions on top of the fish. Sauce the fish.

Sautéed Scallops with Tomato Sauce

SERVES 6

3 garlic cloves
¾ cup olive oil
1½ cups tomato purée
1 tablespoon tomato paste
2 tablespoons finely minced ginger
Salt
Black pepper
Juice of 1 lemon
Juice of 1 orange
2 pounds sea scallops

Mince 2 cloves garlic. Heat ¼ cup oil and sauté minced garlic for 30 seconds over medium heat. Add tomato purée, tomato paste, and ginger. Season with salt and pepper. Stir mixture and let simmer for approximately 5 minutes over medium to low heat. Add lemon and orange juices and simmer for 7 minutes. Strain sauce and set aside. Season scallops with salt and pepper. Crush remaining garlic clove. Heat 2 tablespoons oil and sauté crushed garlic until golden, then remove garlic. Cook scallops in batches over medium-high heat for 3 minutes each side, using remaining oil as needed. Place in large serving dish and drizzle with sauce. Serve hot.

Shrimp Cocktail

Serves 4–6

1 tablespoon salt
2 bay leaves
10 peppercorns
½ cup white wine
Juice of ½ lemon
2 pounds jumbo shrimp (large, under 15), peeled and deveined
3 tablespoons ketchup
2 teaspoons horseradish
½ teaspoon hot pepper sauce

Bring 3 quarts of water to a boil. Add salt, bay leaves, peppercorns, white wine, and lemon juice. When water comes to a boil again, add shrimp. Bring to a boil again, then remove shrimp and plunge into ice water. Drain shrimp and place in serving bowl. To make cocktail sauce, combine ketchup, horseradish, and hot sauce, and serve with the shrimp.

Shrimp Marinara

Serves 4–6

½ cup olive oil
7 garlic cloves, sliced
2 pounds jumbo shrimp, peeled and deveined
One 28-ounce can crushed tomatoes
1 teaspoon crushed red pepper
Salt
Black pepper
3 tablespoons chopped parsley
10 fresh basil leaves, chopped

Sauté garlic in ¼ cup oil until slightly golden. Add shrimp and cook 1 minute each side, being careful not to overcrowd pan. Remove shrimp and to same pan add tomatoes, red pepper, remaining oil, salt, and pepper. Bring to a boil, reduce heat, and simmer 10 minutes, pan partially covered, stirring occasionally. Add shrimp, parsley, and basil. Raise heat and cook for 30 to 45 seconds.

Broiled or Grilled Shrimp with Thyme

SERVES 2–3

11 garlic cloves
½ cup olive oil
1 pound jumbo shrimp, unpeeled, deveined, butterflied
1 tablespoon fresh thyme, chopped
1 teaspoon salt

Crush 10 garlic cloves and combine with oil. Let sit 1 to 2 hours. Strain and discard garlic. Spoon enough of this garlic-infused oil over shrimp to coat. Finely mince 1 clove garlic. Combine garlic, thyme, and salt and marinate shrimp in this mixture for 1 hour in refrigerator. Preheat broiler. Place shrimp cut side down on oiled broiler pan, using 2 tablespoons of garlic-infused oil, and broil 7 minutes; if grilling, grill with the shell for 3 minutes on each side. Discard remaining garlic-infused oil—it poses a botulism risk if stored.

Baked Shrimp Oreganato

SERVES 4–6

8 tablespoons plus 1 teaspoon olive oil
2 pounds jumbo shrimp, peeled, deveined, and butterflied
Salt
Black pepper
1 cup plain bread crumbs
2 tablespoons chopped parsley
2 garlic cloves, finely chopped
3 tablespoons grated Parmesan cheese
1 tablespoon dried oregano

Preheat oven to 400 degrees. Grease a baking dish with 1 teaspoon oil. Season shrimp with salt and pepper and place them cut side up in dish. In a separate bowl, mix bread crumbs, parsley, garlic, cheese, 6 tablespoons olive oil, and oregano. Sprinkle bread crumb mixture over shrimp. Cover dish with foil and bake 10 minutes. Turn oven to broil. Remove foil and broil for 1 minute. Drizzle remaining oil over shrimp and serve immediately.

Roasted Lobster

Serves 1–2

One 3-pound lobster
Juice of 1 lemon
1 teaspoon Dijon mustard
2 teaspoons chopped parsley
1 teaspoon oregano
½ teaspoon salt
½ teaspoon black pepper
5 tablespoons olive oil
2 tablespoons bread crumbs

Preheat oven to 375 degrees. Cut lobster down the middle into halves, holding the lobster by its back and starting at the head. Clean out lobster and place on baking tray shell down. In a small saucepan combine lemon, mustard, parsley, oregano, salt, pepper, and 3 tablespoons oil over low heat for 1 minute. Pour sauce over lobster and top with bread crumbs. Drizzle with remaining oil. Bake 20 to 30 minutes.

Boiled Lobster

Serves 1–2

One 3-pound live lobster
5 cloves
1 onion, quartered
1 tablespoon salt
10 black peppercorns
¼ cup dry white wine
juice of 1 lemon
1 to 2 tablespoons olive oil

In a large pot, bring 6 quarts of water to a boil. Add whole lobster, cloves, onion, salt, peppercorns, lemon juice, and wine. Cook for 20 minutes at a low boil. Turn off heat and let lobster sit in broth until cool. Remove lobster meat, cut into pieces, and drizzle with oil.

Broiled Swordfish

The success of this recipe depends on not turning the fish. Broil on one side only.

Serves 4–6

2 pounds swordfish, 1 inch thick
6 tablespoons olive oil
1 teaspoon salt
1 teaspoon black pepper
Juice of 1½ lemons
1 teaspoon soy sauce
1 garlic clove, crushed
1 teaspoon oregano

Preheat broiler. Brush swordfish with 3 tablespoons oil and season with salt and pepper. Broil 7 to 8 minutes 7 inches from heat source; do not turn fish. Mix remaining oil, lemon juice, soy sauce, garlic, and oregano. Pour over fish and broil 1 minute more.

Swordfish Rollatini

Serves 2–4

1 pound swordfish, sliced into thin pieces 2 inches by 4 inches
6 ounces plain bread crumbs
2 ounces grated Parmesan or Romano cheese
2 tablespoons chopped parsley
1 or 2 garlic cloves, finely minced
Salt
Black pepper
½ cup plus 2 tablespoons olive oil
½ cup dry white wine

Preheat oven to 475 degrees. Pound fish very gently between sheets of plastic wrap and set aside. In a bowl, combine bread crumbs, cheese, parsley, garlic, and salt and pepper to taste. Mix with enough olive oil to maintain shape when squeezed. Let bread crumb mixture rest 20 minutes to soften bread crumbs and blend flavors. Reserve 2 tablespoons oil and pour the rest onto a baking sheet. Place 1 teaspoon stuffing on each fish slice. Roll swordfish and place rolls seam side down on baking sheet. Drizzle with reserved 2 tablespoons oil. Cover tray with foil and bake on lowest rack of oven for 5 minutes. Remove foil, pour wine around fish, and bake uncovered 5 minutes until alcohol cooks off.

Swordfish with Capers

SERVES 6

8 tablespoons olive oil
Six 6-ounce swordfish steaks, 1 inch thick
Salt
Black pepper
3 tablespoons capers, chopped
4 tablespoons chopped parsley
Juice of 2 lemons

Heat 6 tablespoons olive oil in a skillet. Season swordfish with salt and pepper on both sides. Cook swordfish in batches, so as not to overcrowd pan, for approximately 3 minutes on each side. Remove swordfish from pan and keep warm. Add capers and parsley to skillet and remaining 2 tablespoons olive oil. Deglaze with lemon juice. Pour over fish and serve.

Swordfish Kebabs

SERVES 6

1½ pounds swordfish, cut into 1-inch cubes
Salt
Black pepper
1 tablespoon chopped rosemary
Juice and zest of 1 lemon
6 tablespoons olive oil
1 large red onion, cut into chunks
1½ pints cherry tomatoes (approximately 1 pound)

In a large bowl, combine swordfish, salt and pepper to taste, rosemary, lemon juice, lemon zest, and 4 tablespoons olive oil. Mix well with hands and marinate for 15 minutes. Preheat broiler. Oil baking pan with 2 tablespoons olive oil. Thread each skewer with alternating onion, tomato, and fish. Place kebabs on oiled pan and broil 4 inches from heat source 1 to 2 minutes on each side. Do not overcook.

Swordfish alla Stemperata

Serves 6

1½ pounds swordfish cut into 6 slices ½ inch thick
Flour for dredging
6 tablespoons olive oil
1 onion, diced
One 15-ounce can whole peeled tomatoes, crushed by hand
3 tablespoons capers
4 tablespoons green olives, pitted
1 stalk celery, diced
½ cup white vinegar
Salt
Black pepper

Dredge the swordfish in flour and shake off excess. Sauté fish in 4 tablespoons olive oil 1 to 2 minutes on each side; set aside and keep warm. In a clean pan, heat the remaining oil and sauté onion, tomatoes, capers, olives, and celery for 3 to 4 minutes. Add vinegar, salt and pepper to taste, 3 tablespoons water, and cook for 5 minutes. Pour sauce over swordfish and serve hot.

Baked Tilefish

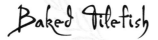

This recipe will also work well with scrod.

Serves 2–3

1 pound tilefish steak, 1 inch thick
4 tablespoons olive oil
1 teaspoon salt
1 teaspoon black pepper
1 large onion, thinly sliced
4 canned plum tomatoes, crushed by hand
½ cup white wine

Preheat oven to 450 degrees. Pour 2 tablespoons oil in large baking pan and add tilefish. Top fish with salt, pepper, onion, and tomatoes and drizzle with 1 tablespoon oil. Pour wine around fish. Cover with foil and bake 25 minutes. Switch oven to broil, remove foil, and broil 2 to 3 minutes. Place fish on serving dish, pour juice over fish, and drizzle with remaining 1 tablespoon oil.

Sweet and Sour Red Snapper

This is a personal favorite of mine. This versatile recipe can also be used with striped sea bass, black sea bass, tilapia, and porgy.

Serves 4–6

2 pounds red snapper filets
Salt
Black pepper
½ cup flour
8 tablespoons olive oil
1 large onion, chopped
1 cup chopped celery
One 8-ounce can tomato sauce
20 green marinated Sicilian olives, pitted and halved
3 tablespoons capers, rinsed
¼ cup sugar
¼ cup white wine vinegar

Season fish with salt and pepper and dredge in flour, shaking off excess. Sauté fish in 5 tablespoons oil for 3 minutes on each side. Remove fish and set aside; discard liquid in pan. Heat remaining 3 tablespoons oil and sauté onion and celery for approximately 5 minutes. Add tomato sauce, olives, and capers. In a small bowl combine sugar and vinegar and add to skillet (some sugar may remain undissolved). Bring to a boil, then reduce heat, cover, and simmer 5 minutes. Return fish to pan, placing on top of sauce, and cook 5 to 10 minutes on low simmer, covered. Spoon sauce on top to serve.

Broiled Red Snapper

SERVES 4–6

One 2-pound red snapper or 2 large filets
3 tablespoons olive oil
1 teaspoon soy sauce
Juice of 1½ lemons
1 teaspoon salt
1 teaspoon black pepper
1 teaspoon oregano
1 garlic clove, finely minced

Preheat broiler. Brush fish with 1 tablespoon olive oil. If using filets, broil for 7 to 8 minutes with skin side up and then 1 to 2 minutes skin side down. If using a whole fish, broil for 10 minutes on each side. For sauce, combine soy sauce, remaining oil, lemon juice, salt, pepper, oregano, and garlic. Pour over fish and broil 1 more minute.

Striped Bass Oreganato

SERVES 1–2

2 pounds striped bass filets, 1 to 1½ inches thick
6 tablespoons olive oil
2 garlic cloves, finely chopped
One 18-ounce can crushed tomatoes
1 tablespoon oregano
1 teaspoon salt
1 teaspoon black pepper
2 tablespoons chopped parsley
3 tablespoons Romano cheese, grated

Preheat oven to 450 degrees. Rub both sides of fish with 3 tablespoons oil. Spread garlic evenly on fish. Cover fish completely with tomatoes. Add oregano, salt, pepper, and parsley. Add grated cheese to top and drizzle remaining oil on top of fish. Bake for 30 to 35 minutes. The house will smell wonderful.

Black Sea Bass in Umido

Serves 4–6

3 tablespoons olive oil
10 garlic cloves, crushed
3 tablespoons chopped parsley
6 tablespoons crushed tomatoes or canned cherry tomatoes
2 pounds sea bass filets (or 1 whole 2-pound fish)
1 teaspoon salt
1 teaspoon black pepper
½ cup white wine

Sauté garlic and parsley in oil for 1 minute. Add tomatoes and cook 3 minutes over medium heat, stirring occasionally. Add fish (if using filets, place skin side down), salt, pepper, and wine. Bring to a boil, reduce heat, and simmer 10 to 12 minutes, covered, without turning fish. For whole fish, turn after 7 minutes and simmer another 7 minutes. Serve with sauce poured over fish. Bread tastes great dunked in the broth.

Whiting in Brodo

Serves 4

3 garlic cloves, crushed
1 tablespoon chopped parsley
4 whiting, cleaned, heads removed, and filleted
6 tablespoons olive oil
1 tablespoon salt
½ teaspoon black pepper

Bring 1 quart of water to a boil. Add garlic, parsley, whiting, 3 tablespoons oil, salt, and pepper. Boil gently for 15 minutes. Serve the fish in the broth, with the remaining oil drizzled on top.

Broiled Branzino

This recipe works well with many other varieties of fish, including striped sea bass, black sea bass, red snapper, and orata.

SERVES 4

One 2-pound branzino, cleaned, scaled, fins removed
4 tablespoons olive oil
1 teaspoon salt
1 teaspoon black pepper
1 teaspoon soy sauce
Juice of 1 lemon
1 large garlic clove, finely minced
½ teaspoon oregano

Preheat broiler. Lightly coat entire fish with 1 tablespoon oil. Broil fish for 6 to 7 minutes on each side. In a separate bowl mix remaining oil, salt, pepper, soy sauce, lemon juice, garlic, and oregano. Pour sauce over the fish and broil for 1 minute. Spoon juices over fish before serving.

Sicilian-Style Calamari

SERVES 2–4

8 garlic cloves
¼ cup plus 3 tablespoons olive oil
One 28-ounce can crushed tomatoes
Salt
¼ cup capers
1 tablespoon crushed red pepper
¼ cup white wine
1½ pounds squid, cleaned, cut into ½-inch rings
5 scallions, thinly sliced
Black pepper

Crush 4 garlic cloves and sauté in 3 tablespoons oil until golden. Add tomatoes and 1 teaspoon salt. Bring to a boil, then reduce heat and simmer for 20 minutes. Set tomato sauce aside. In a sauté pan heat remaining oil over high heat. Thinly slice remaining garlic and add to pan with capers and red pepper. Cook for 2 minutes. Add wine and tomato sauce and bring to a simmer. Add squid, mix well, and simmer another 2 minutes, or until squid is completely opaque. Add scallions and salt and pepper to taste. Note: You can cook calamari for 2 or 20 minutes; anything in between and you will get tough calamari.

Stuffed Calamari

SERVES 2–4

1½ pounds squid, cleaned, tentacles cut off and body (tube) intact
Juice of 1 lemon
4 tablespoons olive oil
1 garlic clove, finely minced
2 anchovies, chopped
1 tablespoon chopped parsley
1 cup bread crumbs
½ teaspoon salt
1 teaspoon black pepper

Preheat oven to 400 degrees. Cook tentacles in 1 quart water with lemon juice 10 to 15 minutes, until tender. Chop tentacles and combine in a bowl with 3 tablespoons oil, garlic, anchovies, parsley, bread crumbs, salt, and pepper. Stuff the bodies with the bread crumb mixture and close the openings with toothpicks. Sprinkle any remaining bread crumb mixture over top. Grease a baking dish with remaining oil and place squid in baking dish. Bake 30 minutes.

Calamari Marinara Fra Diavolo

I frequently have two servings of this for lunch—it's delicious.

SERVES 4–6

3 tablespoons olive oil
8 garlic cloves, crushed
1 teaspoon red pepper flakes
3 pounds squid, cleaned, body separated from tentacles and cut into 2- to 3-inch wedges, tentacles cut in half
One 28-ounce can crushed tomatoes
1 teaspoon salt

Heat oil and sauté garlic and red pepper flakes until garlic is golden. Add squid and sauté, stirring occasionally, for 2 to 3 minutes, with the pan partially covered. Add tomatoes and salt and bring to a boil. Reduce heat and simmer for 20 to 30 minutes, stirring frequently.

Mussels Marinara

Serves 3–6

1 tablespoon olive oil
6 garlic cloves, minced
1 cup chopped onions
One 28-ounce can crushed or diced tomatoes
2 tablespoons lemon juice
½ cup white wine
2 tablespoons chopped parsley
1 tablespoon chopped fresh oregano
3 pounds mussels, scrubbed

In a large pan, heat oil and sauté garlic and onions until onions are translucent. Add tomatoes with the juice, wine, lemon juice, parsley, and oregano and cook 3 to 4 minutes covered. Add mussels and cook approximately 7 to 10 minutes, stirring to ensure that all mussels open. Serve hot.

Mussels with Garlic and Wine

Serves 3–6

2 tablespoons olive oil
5 garlic cloves, sliced
3 pounds mussels, scrubbed
½ cup white wine
½ teaspoon oregano
2 tablespoons chopped parsley

Sauté garlic in olive oil for 30 seconds. Add mussels, wine, oregano, and 1 tablespoon parsley. Cover. As mussels begin to open, stir from the bottom to allow bottom shells to open. Cook until all mussels are open—don't overcook. Add remaining parsley and serve in their own juice.

Steamed Clams

Serves 1

2 tablespoons olive oil
2 garlic cloves, thinly sliced
1–1½ dozen littleneck clams, scrubbed and thoroughly cleaned
¼ cup white wine
2 tablespoons chopped parsley
1 lemon, quartered

In a large pan heat olive oil over medium-high heat. Add garlic and cook until golden, about 30 seconds. Add clams and white wine. Cover and cook over high heat about 2 minutes, stirring until all clams have opened; do not overcook or clams will be rubbery. Sprinkle with parsley. Serve in their own juice with lemon wedges.

ANGELO ACQUISTA, M.D.
NEW YORK, NY 10022
DEA # LIC#

NAME ______ AGE ______
ADDRESS ______ DATE ______
RX ILLEGAL IF NOT SAFETY BLUE BACKGROUND

℞

Poultry

THIS PRESCRIPTION WILL BE FILLED GENERICALLY
UNLESS PRESCRIBER WRITES "d a w" IN THE BOX BELOW.

Refill ______ times

NR ______ Label ______ Dispense As Written BCM

Chicken Cacciatore

This delicious recipe is from Cipriani, New York.

SERVES 6

6 chicken breasts and/or legs, skin removed
Salt
Black pepper
Flour for dredging, plus 1 tablespoon
6 tablespoons olive oil
1 medium onion, chopped
2 celery ribs, chopped
1 carrot, chopped
½ pound white or shiitake mushrooms, chopped
1 garlic clove, finely minced
1 teaspoon chopped fresh thyme
1 teaspoon chopped fresh rosemary
3 plum tomatoes, diced
1 cup white wine
1 cup beef stock

Season chicken pieces with salt and pepper. Dredge seasoned chicken in flour, shaking off excess. Heat 4 tablespoons oil over medium heat and cook chicken in batches until golden brown on both sides, about 15 minutes. Remove chicken and wipe pan clean with paper towels. Add remaining oil, onion, celery, carrot, mushrooms, and garlic to pan. Cook until soft, about 10 minutes. Stir in herbs and tomatoes. Turn up heat and add wine. Boil for 3 to 4 minutes. Reduce heat to medium and sprinkle 1 tablespoon of flour over vegetables. Stir to combine thoroughly and cook 2 to 3 minutes. Add stock and cook, stirring, for another 2 to 3 minutes. Return chicken to pan and spoon some of the vegetable mixture over the chicken. Simmer, partially covered, for 15 minutes, then turn chicken and simmer 15 minutes more.

Chicken with Garlic and Vegetables

This recipe is from Cipriani, New York.

Serves 4

4 teaspoons olive oil
1 to 1½ pounds skinless, boneless chicken breast halves
2 carrots, peeled and cut into thin strips
1 medium leek, white part only, thoroughly washed and cut into thin strips
1 red bell pepper, seeded and cut into thin strips
2 garlic cloves, finely minced
½ cup canned crushed tomatoes
Salt
Black pepper

Heat oil in a large skillet over medium heat. Sauté chicken 4 to 5 minutes per side, until chicken is opaque throughout. Transfer to a platter and keep warm. Add carrots to skillet and sauté over medium heat for 1 minute. Add leek, bell pepper, and garlic. Sauté another minute. Stir in tomatoes. Simmer 2 minutes or until vegetables are tender. Season with salt and pepper. Serve vegetables over chicken.

Chicken Scarpariello

Serve 8–10

4 pounds chicken, cut into 2- to 3-inch pieces
Salt
Black pepper
4 tablespoons olive oil
8 to 12 garlic cloves, finely minced
8 medium-hot cherry peppers, quartered (or non-spicy bottled cherry peppers in vinaigrette)
⅓ cup red wine vinegar
⅓ cup white wine
½ cup chicken stock

Preheat broiler. Season chicken with salt and pepper. Heat 3 tablespoons of oil and sauté chicken until golden brown on all sides, 6 to 7 minutes total. Drain chicken and place in single layer on baking pan. Wipe skillet, add 1 tablespoon oil, and sauté garlic until golden. Add cherry peppers, salt, and pepper, and cook, stirring, for 30 seconds. Add vinegar, bring to a boil, and reduce liquid by half. Add wine and reduce by half again. Add stock and bring to a boil. Pour stock mixture over chicken in baking pan. Place in oven and broil for 5 to 7 minutes, stirring occasionally, until liquid thickens slightly and chicken is cooked through.

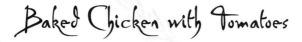

Baked Chicken with Tomatoes

Serves 2–4

1 chicken, about 3 pounds, cut into 14 to 16 pieces
One 14-ounce can crushed tomatoes
3 tablespoons grated Romano cheese
1 tablespoon salt
1 tablespoon black pepper
2 tablespoons olive oil
½ cup white wine

Preheat oven to 400 degrees. In a large baking dish place chicken in a single layer. Top with tomatoes, cheese, salt, and pepper. Drizzle with oil. Pour wine around chicken. Bake 40 to 45 minutes. Turn oven to broil and broil 3 minutes.

Broiled Chicken

Serves 1–3

1 teaspoon salt
1 teaspoon black pepper
1 tablespoon chopped parsley
¼ cup olive oil
Juice of 1 lemon
1 tablespoon red wine vinegar
1 teaspoon oregano
2 garlic cloves, chopped
½ chicken (with bones), cut into 4 to 6 pieces, skin on

In large bowl combine salt, pepper, parsley, oil, half the lemon juice, vinegar, oregano, and garlic; add chicken, mix, and marinate in the refrigerator for 1 to 2 hours. Preheat broiler. Remove the chicken and broil 30 minutes on lowest oven rack until first side is brown. Turn and broil 20 minutes until brown and cooked through. Remove the skin. Squeeze remaining lemon juice over and serve with pan juices.

Broiled Chicken with Garlic and Lime

Serves 1–3

6 garlic cloves, finely minced
1 tablespoon salt
2 tablespoons pepper
3 tablespoons lime juice
½ chicken with the skin, cut into 4 pieces

Combine garlic, salt, pepper, and lime juice, and rub chicken with the mixture. Marinate in refrigerator for 1 to 2 hours. Preheat broiler. Broil (or grill) 30 minutes, turning chicken as needed, until chicken is no longer pink inside. Remove skin before eating.

Broiled Chicken with Orange and Lime

Serves 4–6

2 pounds chicken breast, skin on
3 garlic cloves, crushed
Juice of 1 orange
Juice of 1 lime
1 teaspoon salt
1 teaspoon black pepper

Combine all ingredients and marinate in refrigerator for 30 minutes. Preheat broiler. Remove chicken from marinade and broil skin side down 7 to 9 minutes. Turn chicken over and broil for 7 minutes more or until done. Remove skin before serving.

Broiled Chicken with Balsamic Vinegar

Serves 4–6

2 pounds skinless, boneless chicken breast
½ cup chicken stock
1 teaspoon salt
1 teaspoon black pepper
1 tablespoon dry mustard
2 tablespoons sugar
4 garlic cloves, chopped
1 cup balsamic vinegar
2 tablespoons Dijon mustard

Mix all ingredients in a large bowl, cover, and marinate in refrigerator 8 hours, turning chicken occasionally. Preheat broiler. Remove chicken from marinade and broil (or grill) about 5 to 7 minutes on each side, basting chicken with marinade while cooking.

Broiled Chicken with Lemon

Serves 4–6

1 bay leaf
1 cup chicken stock
2 tablespoons fresh oregano
¼ cup olive oil
½ cup freshly squeezed lemon juice
1 teaspoon salt
2 pounds boneless chicken breast with skin

In bowl, combine all ingredients and marinate in refrigerator for 1 to 2 hours. Remove chicken from marinade. Preheat broiler. Broil chicken for 5 to 7 minutes on each side. Remove skin before serving.

ANGELO ACQUISTA, M.D.
NEW YORK, NY 10022
DEA # LIC#

NAME ______ AGE ______
ADDRESS ______ DATE ______
RX ILLEGAL IF NOT SAFETY BLUE BACKGROUND

Rx

Meat

THIS PRESCRIPTION WILL BE FILLED GENERICALLY
UNLESS PRESCRIBER WRITES "d a w" IN THE BOX BELOW.

Refill ______ times
NR ______ Label ______ Dispense As Written BCM

Filet Mignon

This is a great, simple dish to make. I often prepare a larger version of this, 6 to 8 pounds, when I have a lot of guests and little time.

SERVES 4

1 tablespoon salt
1 tablespoon black pepper
1 tablespoon thyme
2 garlic cloves, chopped
2 tablespoons olive oil
2 pounds filet mignon in one piece

In a small bowl, combine salt, pepper, thyme, garlic, and olive oil. With a small knife, make 8 to 10 slits in the meat and rub the spice mixture into the slits and over the surface. Let meat sit for 30 minutes to 1 hour in the refrigerator. Remove from refrigerator and let sit at room temperature 30 minutes. Preheat oven to 475 degrees and roast meat for 20 to 30 minutes, or until the internal temperature reaches 120 degrees for rare and 130 to 135 degrees for medium. Remove from oven and let meat rest for 5 to 10 minutes before slicing.

Veal Piccata

SERVES 2–4

1 pound veal cutlets, cut ¼-inch thick, pounded thin
Salt
Black pepper
½ cup flour for dredging
4 tablespoons olive oil
½ cup chicken stock
¼ cup lemon juice
1 tablespoon butter or trans-fat-free margarine (optional)
1 tablespoon chopped parsley

Season veal with salt and pepper and dredge in flour, shaking off the excess. In a large skillet, heat 2 tablespoons oil over medium-high heat and cook veal in batches (adding more oil as needed), 2 minutes per side, keeping cooked cutlets warm in a 200-degree oven. Pour off oil and add chicken stock and lemon juice to pan. Boil for 1 minute. Remove from heat and blend in butter. Add parsley and pour sauce over meat.

Veal Cutlet Pizzaiola

Serves 2–4

1½ pounds veal cutlets, cut ¼-inch thick, pounded thin
Salt
Black pepper
1 cup flour
6 tablespoons olive oil
½ cup chicken stock
1 tablespoon butter or trans-fat-free margarine (optional)
3 tablespoons chopped parsley
⅓ cup tomato sauce or Mom's Quick Tomato Sauce, page 227, heated

Season veal with salt and pepper and dredge in flour, shaking off excess. In a large skillet, heat 2 tablespoons oil over medium-high heat and cook veal in batches (adding oil as needed), 2 minutes per side, keeping cooked cutlets warm in a 200-degree oven. Pour off oil. Add chicken stock to skillet and boil 1 minute. Remove from heat and whisk in butter. Add parsley. Drizzle hot tomato sauce and pan juices over the veal. Serve right away.

Veal Stew

Serves 4–6

2 pounds boneless veal from the shoulder, cut into 1- to 2-inch pieces
Salt
Black pepper
1 cup flour for dredging
¼ cup olive oil
1 medium onion, chopped
2 celery stalks, chopped
2 garlic cloves, chopped
½ cup wine
2 cups tomato sauce

Season veal with salt and pepper and dredge in flour, shaking off excess. Heat oil over medium heat and brown veal in batches. Return meat to pan and add onions, celery, and garlic. Cook, stirring, for 2 minutes. Add wine, bring to a boil, and cook 2 minutes more. Reduce heat, add tomato sauce, cover, and simmer for 1½ hours, until meat is tender, stirring occasionally and adding warm water if sauce thickens too much.

Veal Marsala

This dish is normally prepared with butter. I use extra-virgin olive oil and accept the fact that the sauce will not be as thick, velvety, and rich. The taste is still great, and there's less animal fat. Whenever you flour meat, flour it just before you are ready to cook it. Doing it in advance will make the meat soggy.

SERVES 4–6

1½ pounds veal cutlets, cut ¼-inch thick, pounded thin
Salt
Black pepper
1 cup flour for dredging
½ cup olive oil
3 cups mushrooms, cleaned, thinly sliced
½ cup Marsala wine
1 cup chicken stock
2 tablespoons chopped parsley

Season veal with salt and pepper and dredge in flour, shaking off excess. In a large skillet, heat 2 tablespoons oil over medium heat and cook veal in batches (adding oil as needed), about 2 minutes each side, keeping cooked cutlets warm in a 200-degree oven. Wipe pan of old oil and add 2 tablespoons fresh oil. Sauté mushrooms with salt and pepper for 3 to 4 minutes, until mushrooms begin to brown, allowing water from mushrooms to evaporate. Add Marsala and boil 2 minutes. Add chicken stock and reduce liquid by half. Return veal to skillet and spoon juice and mushrooms over the meat. Add parsley and cook until meat is heated through, and serve in a warm dish.

Broiled Lamb Chops

This is an easy dish that will add variety to your menu. Have this with an arugula and onion salad, steamed or sautéed broccoli rabe, and a glass of red wine. If you don't have time to make the garlic-rosemary oil, just season lamb chops with a little lemon, salt, and pepper, and you're ready to eat in 10 minutes.

Serves 3–4

¼ cup olive oil
2 to 3 sprigs rosemary
4 garlic cloves, crushed
Salt
Black pepper
10 rib or loin lamb chops, 1 to 1¼ inches thick

In a small saucepan, heat oil and rosemary for 2 to 3 minutes. Remove from heat and add garlic. Let sit for 1 to 2 hours. Preheat broiler. Brush oil mixture on both sides of lamb and season with salt and pepper. Broil (or grill) 3 to 5 minutes on each side and serve immediately.

Roast Leg of Lamb

Serves 6–8

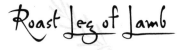

4 garlic cloves, finely minced
1 teaspoon salt
1 teaspoon black pepper
2 tablespoons chopped fresh rosemary
2 tablespoons olive oil
¼ cup Dijon mustard
One 6–8 pound leg of lamb, bone-in, trimmed of excess fat

Preheat oven to 350 degrees. In a bowl, combine garlic, salt, pepper, rosemary, olive oil, and Dijon mustard. Brush mixture on lamb. Roast lamb 1 hour 15 minutes for medium (internal temperature 130 degrees). Let the roast rest for 20 minutes before cutting and serving.

Roasted Pork Loin

Serves 6–8

4 pounds boneless pork loin
2 tablespoons olive oil
1 tablespoon coarse salt
1 tablespoon garlic powder
1 tablespoon dried thyme
1 tablespoon black pepper
1 tablespoon parsley flakes

Rub pork with olive oil. Combine salt, garlic powder, thyme, pepper, and parsley and rub over pork. Let meat sit in refrigerator 2 hours or up to overnight. Preheat oven to 350 degrees. Place pork, fat side up, in a shallow roasting pan and cook for 1 hour and 15 minutes or until internal temperature reaches 145 degrees. Remove pork from the oven, cover loosely with foil, and allow to rest for 20 minutes. The internal temperature will continue to rise to approximately 150 degrees. Cut into ¼-inch-thick slices.

Rib Roast

This recipe is healthiest if you use a lean cut of rib roast.

Serves 6–8

2 heads of garlic (about 30 cloves)
3 tablespoons olive oil
⅓ cup bottled white horseradish
½ teaspoon coarse salt
4- to 6-pound boneless rib roast

Preheat oven to 350 degrees. Slice off the top of the garlic heads and drizzle with oil. Roast garlic until soft, about 30 minutes. Squeeze the roasted cloves into a small food processor, adding any olive oil that remains in the pan. Add the horseradish and salt and purée. Spread the mixture over the rib roast and refrigerate for 3 hours or up to overnight. Roast at 350 degrees for 1½ hours or until internal temperature reaches 125 to 130 degrees for medium. Let meat rest before serving.

ANGELO ACQUISTA, M.D.
NEW YORK, NY 10022
DEA # LIC#

NAME ______ AGE ______
ADDRESS ______ DATE ______
RX ILLEGAL IF NOT SAFETY BLUE BACKGROUND

Rx

Desserts

THIS PRESCRIPTION WILL BE FILLED GENERICALLY
UNLESS PRESCRIBER WRITES "d a w" IN THE BOX BELOW.

Refill ______ times
NR ______ Label ______ Dispense As Written BCM

Sandro's Mixed Berries with Balsamic Vinegar and Grand Marnier

Serves 6–8

4 heaping tablespoons plus ½ cup sugar
Peel of 1 orange, all white pith removed, cut into 12 pieces
½ cup orange juice
1 tablespoon balsamic vinegar
2 pints blueberries
2 pints strawberries, hulled and quartered
2 tablespoons Grand Marnier

Place 4 heaping tablespoons of sugar and 3 tablespoons water in a sauté pan and cook over high heat until caramelized. Add the orange peel, orange juice, and balsamic vinegar. Cook 1 minute, strain, and discard orange peel. Heat a separate large sauté pan over very high heat. Mix berries and ½ cup sugar and add to hot pan. Add caramelized sugar mixture and cook 1 to 2 minutes. Add Grand Marnier and remove from heat. The sauce can be refrigerated for months.

Poached Pears in Chianti

Serves 6

1 bottle Chianti wine
2 cups port wine
3 cinnamon sticks
Juice and zest of ½ lemon
1 cup sugar
6 Bosc pears, peeled

Bring Chianti, port, cinnamon sticks, lemon juice, lemon zest, and sugar to a boil in a saucepan. Add the peeled pears and poach for 20 to 30 minutes. Remove the pears and discard the cinnamon sticks and the lemon zest. Reduce liquid by cooking for an additional 10 minutes or until it thickens. Pour reduced liquid through a strainer. Serve pears with reduced liquid drizzled over top.

ANGELO ACQUISTA, M.D.

NEW YORK, NY 10022

DEA # LIC#

NAME ______ AGE ______

ADDRESS ______ DATE ______

RX ILLEGAL IF NOT SAFETY BLUE BACKGROUND

℞

Snacks

THIS PRESCRIPTION WILL BE FILLED GENERICALLY
UNLESS PRESCRIBER WRITES "d a w" IN THE BOX BELOW.

Refill ______ times

NR ______ Label ______ Dispense As Written BCM

SNACKS ARE A GREAT WAY TO CURB HUNGER AND ENCOURAGE THE THERMIC effect (burning calories from the digestion of food), as well as to satisfy all of your healthy servings from the Mediterranean Prescription pyramid. My favorite snacks are nuts; dried fruits like apricots and prunes; grapes; orange slices; and—best of all—a combination of a few of the above at a time. I snack on these foods several times a day—to me there are no snacks more filling or delicious. Be sure to count your snacks as a part of your daily allotment of foods.

Great Mediterranean Snacks

- Fresh fruit of any kind
- Dried fruit such as raisins, figs, apricots, dates, currants, cherries, and blueberries (about 2 tablespoons)
- Fresh vegetables of any kind

- Fresh cut vegetables with any of the following dips:
  Hummus (which comes in many delicious varieties)
  Low-fat salad dressing
  Low-fat cottage cheese
  Low-fat ricotta cheese
  Eggplant spread
  Bean dip
  Olive oil drizzled over (could also sprinkle grated cheese or red pepper flakes on top)

- Whole-wheat pita bread with any of the dips above; toast the bread first if you like and break it into chips

- A slice of whole-wheat bread, pita bread, or English muffin with a touch of olive oil drizzled over it and 1 ounce part-skim mozzarella cheese on top, microwaved for about 25 seconds or baked in toaster oven for 1 minute to melt cheese; could also add fresh tomato or a tablespoon or two of tomato sauce underneath the cheese

- Bruschetta, made with toasted whole-wheat Italian bread topped with tomato sauce, chopped vegetables, and/or grated cheese

- Tomatoes mixed with low-fat cottage cheese with a dash of salt and pepper

- Celery sticks with hummus, almond butter, or peanut butter (non-hydrogenated) on top

- Salad (but leave off the high-fat cheeses and cream-based salad dressings); try sprinkling canned chickpeas or pine nuts over it

- Low-calorie soup, such as any vegetable soup that's not cream-based

- Roasted beans

- A handful of nuts (about 2 tablespoons)

- A handful of sunflower or pumpkin seeds (about 2 tablespoons)

- Low-calorie yogurt; try mixing it with fruit and/or granola

- Sorbet or sugar-free sorbet

- Pickles

- Water with a lemon wedge (sometimes that's all it takes to quell your hunger)

ANGELO ACQUISTA, M.D.
NEW YORK, NY 10022
DEA # LIC#

NAME AGE
ADDRESS DATE
RX ILLEGAL IF NOT SAFETY BLUE BACKGROUND

℞

Dressings and Sauces

THIS PRESCRIPTION WILL BE FILLED GENERICALLY
UNLESS PRESCRIBER WRITES "d a w" IN THE BOX BELOW.

Refill .... times

NR ___ Label ___ Dispense As Written BCM

Tomato Base

1 large onion, chopped
2 tablespoons olive oil
One 12-ounce can tomato sauce

Over very low heat, sauté onion in oil for 30 to 40 minutes, covered, stirring occasionally and being careful not to burn onion (you may add 1 tablespoon of water to prevent burning). Add tomato sauce and simmer covered for another 30 minutes, stirring occasionally. This sauce takes a little time to prepare, but it's worth it for the wonderful taste.

Mom's Quick Tomato Sauce

¼ cup olive oil
½ teaspoon red pepper flakes
1 medium onion, chopped
6 garlic cloves, crushed
One 28-ounce can crushed tomatoes
½ teaspoon salt

Heat oil over medium-low heat and sauté red pepper flakes, onion, and garlic about 4 minutes, covered. Add tomatoes and salt. Bring to a boil, lower heat, and simmer partially covered for 20 minutes, stirring occasionally.

Champagne Salad Dressing

Tastes great over mixed greens or iceberg lettuce hearts (take one head of iceberg lettuce and quarter).

Serves 4

3 tablespoons champagne vinegar
½ cup olive oil
1 tablespoon Dijon mustard
¼ teaspoon black pepper
½ teaspoon kosher salt
Pinch of sugar
4 ounces crumbled bleu cheese (optional)

Mix ingredients. If preparing with bleu cheese, use in half when you combine the other ingredients, and sprinkle the rest over salad after you pour dressing over salad greens.

Simple Red Wine Vinaigrette

A very simple yet delightfully fresh taste—tastes great with crunchy salad greens.

Serves 6

3 tablespoons red wine vinegar
½ cup olive oil
Kosher salt to taste

Toss salad with red wine vinegar, then toss with olive oil, then toss again with about two large pinches of salt.

Mediterranean Salad Dressing

Serves 4

½ cup olive oil
Juice of 1 lemon
1 clove garlic, finely minced
½ teaspoon Dijon mustard
Pinch of sugar
Kosher salt
Black pepper
1 tablespoon Kalamata olive juice (optional)

Mix all ingredients. This is best if you let it sit for 5 to 15 minutes before serving to let the garlic infuse into the oil.

Appendix A

The Health Effects of Being Overweight and Obese

People who are overweight or obese are at risk of developing one or more serious medical conditions, which can result in a poor quality of life and even lead to premature death. Excess weight affects virtually every organ system of the human body. Obesity is associated with more than thirty medical conditions, and scientific evidence has established a strong relationship with at least fifteen of those conditions; preliminary data also show the impact of obesity on various other conditions. If you're overweight or obese, losing 10 percent of your starting weight can improve many if not most weight-related medical conditions.

THE HEART AND CIRCULATION

Disorders of the heart and circulation affected by overweight and obesity:
Congestive heart failure
Coronary artery disease (cardiovascular disease)/atherosclerosis
Heart attack

Arrhythmias
Sudden cardiac death
Peripheral vascular disease and peripheral artery disease
High blood pressure (hypertension)
Stroke
Deep vein thrombosis
Chronic venous insufficiency

HEART DISEASE AND STROKE ARE THE FIRST AND THIRD LEADING CAUSES OF death in the United States and together account for more than 35 percent of all deaths. Almost a million Americans die of cardiovascular disease *each year,* which amounts to about one death every thirty seconds. But considering deaths alone understates the overwhelming burden of cardiovascular disease: about sixty-one million Americans (almost one-fourth of the population) live with this disease, which can be debilitating. Heart disease is a leading cause of disability among working adults and is the cause of almost six million hospitalizations every year.

Overweight and obesity play a big part in escalating the risk of illness and death associated with cardiovascular disease. If you have too much fat on your body—and especially if a lot of it is located at your waist—you are at higher risk for such health problems as high blood pressure, high cholesterol, and diabetes. This in turn increases your risk for heart disease. New evidence suggests that by accumulating in heart cells, excess fat directly decreases heart function as well. It is important to note, however, that if you are overweight, even modest weight loss can lower your risk dramatically.

Congestive Heart Failure

Congestive heart failure (also called cardiac failure, cardiac insufficiency, and myocardial insufficiency) is defined as inadequacy of the heart such that it fails to maintain the circulation of blood, which results in a backup or slowdown in the movement of blood and fluids through the circulatory system. Fluids then accumulate in the tissues, and a struggling heart can balloon to twice its normal size. It affects four million to eight million Americans and is the leading cause of hospitalization for people over sixty-five years of age. What's more, the numbers appear to be increasing: from 1979 to 1999, hospitalizations for congestive heart failure rose 155 percent. In a recent study, the lifetime risk for developing it was estimated to be an alarming one in five for both men and women.

Congestive heart failure causes extreme weakness and fatigue. Fluids accumulate in the legs, ankles, and feet most commonly, and can also accumulate around the lungs, liver, and abdomen. It also causes shortness of breath. When heart failure is advanced, Cheyne-Stokes respiration develops, in which a person will breathe rapidly and deeply, then more slowly, then not at all for several seconds. Another possible result of severe disease is the formation of blood clots. These clots may break loose, travel through the body, and block an artery elsewhere. If an artery is blocked by a clot in the brain, a stroke may result.

Overweight and obese men and women have similar elevated risks for congestive heart failure. Approximately 11 percent of cases of heart failure among men and 14 percent among women are attributable to obesity alone. There are several plausible mechanisms that suggest a causal relation between increased body mass index (BMI) and congestive heart failure. Increased BMI is a risk factor for high blood pressure, diabetes, and altered lipid ratios such as high cholesterol (dyslipidemia), all of which augment the risk of heart attack, an important precursor to congestive heart failure. Furthermore, diabetes and hypertension on their own increase the risk of congestive heart failure. Additional literature raises the possibility of a harmful direct effect of fat on heart muscle tissue in animal models of obesity.

Coronary Artery Disease (Cardiovascular Disease)/ Atherosclerosis

Coronary artery disease is almost always due to the buildup of cholesterol and other fatty materials in the blood vessels that supply the heart (the coronary arteries). The accumulation, called atherosclerosis, causes narrowing of those arteries, reducing heart function, and may result in a complete blockage. Coronary artery disease may lead to chest pain (angina), abnormal heart rhythms, blood clots, stroke, heart attack, congestive heart failure, and cardiac arrest.

Coronary artery disease is present in many people who have no symptoms at all (though they may develop symptoms in the future). When it causes symptoms, they can be mild and subtle or sudden and devastating. In one-half of the population, the first recognized symptom of coronary artery disease is a heart attack; in nearly one-half of these patients, the first heart attack is fatal. Coronary heart disease accounts for more than 650,000 deaths per year in the United States, including more than 25 percent of deaths in people older than thirty-five. Cardiovascular disease claims more than three times as many lives as all forms of cancer combined. It is so prevalent that the presence of obstructive coronary artery disease at autopsy approaches 50 percent in elderly women and 70 to 80 percent in elderly men.

Overweight and obesity are strongly linked to the risk of coronary artery disease, particularly when fat is stored in the abdomen. Obesity increases coronary artery disease risk due to its effect on blood lipid levels: excess weight causes a rise in triglycerides and LDL ("bad") cholesterol and lowers HDL ("good") cholesterol. Excess weight may also enhance risk by producing an inflammatory state in the arteries that promotes clogging of the arteries. Excess fat is also associated with diabetes and increased blood pressure, which are risk factors by themselves for coronary artery disease. In addition to causing coronary artery disease, overweight and obesity increase the risk of illness and death associated with coronary heart disease. It is also of note that the effects of obesity on cardiovascular health can begin in childhood, which increases the risk of developing coronary artery disease as an adult.

Heart Attack

A heart attack (also known as myocardial infarction, coronary occlusion, and coronary thrombosis) is the rapid death of heart muscle tissue caused by an inadequate supply of oxygen-rich blood. It is almost always caused by a blockage in a coronary artery (a blood vessel wrapped around the heart that delivers blood to heart muscle), which greatly reduces or cuts off the blood supply to an area of the heart. Once it begins, a window of around three to six hours exists in which to receive treatment and prevent permanent or fatal damage to the heart. Though a heart attack happens suddenly, it is customarily a result of coronary artery disease that has been present for years.

More than 1.1 million people have a heart attack each year in the United States, about two-thirds of whom are men. Approximately 500,000 to 700,000 heart attack patients die; more than half of them die before they can even reach a hospital, and another 10 percent of these deaths occur in the first year after the attack. There are many risks related to gender, age, ethnicity, weight, family history, and lifestyle. It is extremely important to recognize your personal risks for experiencing a heart attack, since more than half of all heart attacks occur without prior symptoms.

The influence of excess weight on the risk of heart attack is significant and essentially the same as it is for coronary artery disease, since the latter usually precedes the former (see page 231).

Arrhythmias

Arrhythmias are abnormal, irregular beats of the heart. The heart usually beats at a steady rate of around 60 to 100 beats per minute, though the rate naturally varies with age, fitness, exercise, and stimuli such as anxiety or excitement. Arrhythmias include conditions where the heart beats too slowly, too fast, irregularly, or with an early beat ("skipped beats"). They occur commonly in middle-aged and older people. In the large majority of cases, arrhythmias are not dangerous in and of themselves, but in some cases they can be very serious and can lead to sudden coronary death.

Because being overweight and obese contributes to the development of certain conditions and diseases that cause arrhythmias, it is an indirect promoter of irregular heart rhythms. The following conditions raise the risk of arrhythmia and are associated with excess weight:

- Congestive heart failure
- Coronary artery disease
- Heart attack
- High blood pressure (hypertension)
- High levels of cholesterol and other fats in the blood
- Diabetes
- Sleep apnea (interrupted breathing during sleep)

In some studies, obesity has been directly linked to certain kinds of arrhythmias even if patients did not have obesity-related conditions such as hypertension or diabetes.

Sudden Cardiac Death

Sudden cardiac death occurs when the heart stops abruptly (cardiac arrest). It can occur minutes after symptoms appear. Most of the cardiac arrests that lead to sudden death occur when the electrical impulses in a diseased heart become rapid and/or chaotic. This irregular heart rhythm (arrhythmia) can cause the heart to suddenly stop beating and pumping blood. If cardiac arrest victims receive no treatment, brain damage can start to occur just four to six minutes after the heart stops pumping blood and getting oxygen to the brain.

All known heart diseases can lead to cardiac arrest and sudden cardiac death. In 80 percent of adult victims of sudden cardiac death, coronary artery disease is present, and two or more major coronary arteries are narrowed by fatty buildups. Scarring from a prior heart attack is found in two-thirds of victims. Because excess weight is a risk factor for the majority of acquired heart conditions, overweight and obesity are significant risk factors for sudden cardiac death as well.

Sudden death from cardiac arrest is a major health problem that has received much less publicity than heart attack and other conditions. In the United States it accounts for around four hundred thousand deaths per year—more deaths than are attributable to lung cancer, breast cancer, or AIDS. In addition, although the direct medical costs are much less than for lingering illnesses, its economic, social, and personal impacts are huge. Sudden cardiac death occurs on average at about sixty years of age, claims many people during their most productive years, and devastates unprepared families.

Peripheral Vascular Disease and Peripheral Artery Disease

Peripheral vascular disease refers to diseases of blood vessels outside the heart and brain. It's often expressed as a narrowing of vessels that carry blood to the legs, arms, stomach, or kidneys. Organic peripheral vascular diseases are caused by structural changes in the blood vessels, such as inflammation and tissue damage; an example is peripheral artery disease, which is caused by fatty buildups in arteries, blocking normal blood flow.

Peripheral artery disease is a condition similar to coronary artery disease in which fatty deposits build up in the inner linings of the artery walls. These blockages restrict blood circulation, mainly in arteries leading to the kidneys, stomach, arms, legs, and feet. In the disease's early stages a common symptom is cramping or fatigue in the legs and buttocks during activity. People with peripheral artery disease also often have fatty buildup in the arteries of the heart and brain. Because of this association, most people with this condition have a higher risk of death from heart attack and stroke.

The good news is that many people with peripheral artery disease can be treated with lifestyle changes. Some of the lifestyle changes to lower your risk include:

- Maintaining a normal weight
- Stopping smoking
- Controlling diabetes (which can be helped by losing weight if you have type 2)
- Controlling high blood pressure (which can be helped by losing weight)
- Being physically active
- Eating a low-saturated-fat, low-cholesterol diet

High Blood Pressure (Hypertension)

Blood pressure is the pressure of the blood within the arteries in the body. It is maintained by the contraction of the left ventricle of the heart, the resistance of certain blood vessels (arterioles and capillaries), the elasticity of the walls of the arteries, and the viscosity and volume of the blood. Blood pressure is gauged by measuring the temporary increase in pressure in the arteries when the heart pumps (systolic pressure) and the pressure when the heart relaxes between beats (diastolic pressure). Readings of systolic/diastolic pressure of 80/50 to 130/85 mmHg are generally considered normal, but what is normal for any individual can vary.

When blood pressure is abnormally high (hypertension), the blood is under greater pressure in the arteries and is flowing through the vessels at a faster rate. Over time, this can cause damage to the inner walls of the blood vessels and provide fertile ground for atherosclerosis to set in (lipid deposits that cause narrowing of the arteries).

Weight or body mass index (BMI) in association with age is the strongest indicator of blood pressure in humans. In fact, over 75 percent of hypertension cases are reported to be directly attributed to obesity. The association between obesity and high blood pressure has been observed in virtually all societies, ages, ethnic groups, and in both genders. The risk of developing hypertension is five to six times greater in obese Americans ages twenty to forty-five compared to nonobese individuals of the same age.

Stroke

See page 237.

Deep Vein Thrombosis

Deep vein thrombosis is the formation of blood clots in certain veins of the leg. Its major complication is pulmonary embolism (a blood clot that breaks off from a vein and travels to the lungs, preventing blood from reaching the lungs). It is estimated that four hundred thousand deaths per year occur as a result of pulmonary embolism; most are not diagnosed until autopsy. Sudden death is often the first and only sign of deep vein thrombosis and pulmonary embolism, with most deaths occurring within the first thirty minutes. Most fatal pulmonary embolisms occur in patients presenting with several risk factors for venous clot formation, one of them being obesity.

Fatalities occurring from pulmonary embolism are a classic example of people and doctors not making the connection between death and the cause of death. When relatives are asked what an individual died of, they simply say he or she died of a blood clot to the lungs. In reality, the individual died of obesity, which caused the blood clot to form in the veins of the leg and travel to the lungs.

Chronic Venous Insufficiency

Chronic venous insufficiency is inadequate blood flow through the veins, causing blood to pool in the veins of the lower legs. Physical manifestations of the condition include varicose veins, leg discomfort (described as pain, pressure, burning, itching, dull ache, or heaviness in the affected part of the leg), nonhealing ulcers (typically at the ankles), swelling of the legs (edema), and skin thickening and altered pigmentation of the legs. It is a common condition, affecting 2 to 5 percent of Americans. Patients tend to be older, sedentary, and obese.

THE BRAIN

Disorders of the brain affected by overweight and obesity:
Stroke*
Cognitive function*
Parkinson's disease*
Depression*
Bipolar disorder*
Hypochondria
Hysteria
Social isolation
Anxiety
Dementia as a result of stroke
Alzheimer's disease
Attention deficit disorder*

* Described below

Stroke

Stroke is defined as the death of brain tissue resulting from the interruption of blood flow to the brain. Stroke can be caused either by a clot obstructing the flow of blood to the brain (ischemic stroke) or by a blood vessel rupturing and preventing blood flow to the brain (hemorrhagic stroke). Within ten seconds after blood flow ceases, brain tissue failure begins, causing brain dysfunction that may evolve to the death of brain tissue if blood flow is not restored within a matter of minutes. Unfortunately, once a stroke is complete, for the most part the neurological deficit (paralysis) is permanent. Because stroke, the leading cause of long-term disability and morbidity and the third leading cause of death in the United States, has few effective therapies, identifying and managing potential risk factors such as elevated BMI remain of great importance.

There are multiple modifiable risk factors that increase the risk of stroke, some important ones being weight gain, elevated body mass index (BMI), and obesity. In a recently published study of twenty-one thousand male doctors followed for twelve and a half years, it was found that increasing BMI was associated with a steady increase in the risk of stroke, independent of the effects of hypertension, diabetes, and cholesterol. In general, a BMI greater than 27 and an elevated waist-to-hip ratio predisposes a person to stroke. Some studies say that waist-to-hip ratio is an even better predictor than BMI.

Cognitive Function

Obesity has been found to decrease cognitive performance as measured by learning, memory, executive functioning, and abstract reasoning in men. It has been found that obese men performed more poorly than men classified as nonobese. The same was not found among women.

Parkinson's Disease

Parkinson's disease is a syndrome that consists of a variable combination of tremor, muscle rigidity, slow movement, and a characteristic disturbance in posture and gait. It is a chronic and progressive disease that typically begins in middle or late life and leads to progressive disability over time. The cause of Parkinson's disease is unknown but may be related to exposure to an unrecognized toxin. Because of the brain's limited ability to regenerate itself, it is more vulnerable than some other organs to permanent disease and chemical injury.

Obesity is associated as a risk factor for chemical- and possibly disease-induced degeneration of brain cells. For example, obese mice show enhanced damage to nerve cells compared to lean mice when exposed to toxins, and data would suggest that the severity of a neurological disease state may be exacerbated by a prior or current obese condition. In addition, recent studies in humans have linked patterns of adiposity (fat accumulation) at midlife with the development of Parkinson's disease. An increase in triceps skinfold thickness, a measure of body fat, has been shown to be associated with the development of Parkinson's disease.

Depression

Depression is defined as depressed mood on a daily basis for a minimum duration of two weeks. Symptoms include change in the patterns of sleep, appetite, and weight; fatigue; impairment in concentration and decision making; feelings of guilt or shame; and thoughts of death or dying. Such patients have a loss of pleasure in all normally enjoyable activities. Approximately 15 percent of the population experiences a major depressive episode at some point in life.

In some research it has been found that a significant association exists between depression and body mass index (BMI). However, a recent study in *Psychiatry Research* showed that abdominal obesity in men, measured by increased waist-to-hip ratio, correlated well with depression and anxiety, while BMI correlated comparatively weakly. Hence depressive symptoms may be more closely related to centralization of body fat stores than to obesity per se. The mechanism for this may be related to increased levels of the hormone cortisol, which is known to lead to the accumulation of fat centrally.

Fish oils (omega-3 fatty acids, available from fatty fish such as mackerel, salmon, and tuna) seem to have a beneficial effect on mood and behavior. For example, university students were less aggressive if they had been fed fish oil for three months; depressed people with high omega-3 levels became less gloomy; manic-depressives on fish oil tend to feel better; and violent offenses among young British prisoners fed fish oil fell by 40 percent. Unlike many other supplements, fish oil supplements do seem to provide benefits similar to those seen from eating the fish themselves.

Bipolar Disorder

Bipolar disorder is common, affecting approximately three million people in the United States, but it is often difficult to diagnose. It is characterized by unpredictable swings in mood from mania to a low of depression. Some of these patients suffer only from recurrent attacks of mania, which is associated with social extroversion, impaired judgment, decreased need for sleep, grandiosity, and at times irritable mood. In severe mania, patients may experience delusions and sometimes paranoid ideation, making the condition difficult to distinguish from schizophrenia. Mood fluctuations are chronic and need to be present for at least two years before the diagnosis is made.

The prevalence of obesity in patients with bipolar disorder greatly exceeds that found in the general population. Obese patients have been found to experience a greater number of lifetime depressive and manic episodes, present with more severe and difficult-to-treat symptoms, and be more likely to develop a depressive recurrence. Obesity may contribute to the severity of bipolar disorder through several factors, including its negative impact on general physical well-being and functioning, quality of life, self-esteem, and psychological well-being. Obesity also contributes to sleep apnea, which may disrupt sleep and other circadian rhythms, thus causing or contributing to mood destabilization.

Attention Deficit/Hyperactivity Disorder

Attention deficit/hyperactivity disorder (ADHD, sometimes still called ADD) is present in 5 to 15 percent of school-age children. Persistence of ADHD into adulthood has been shown to occur in 30 to 50 percent of childhood cases. Adults with a history of ADHD in childhood have greater difficulty functioning compared to their non-ADHD peers. One example of this is the higher rate of substance abuse in ADHD adults compared to the general population; such use is viewed as a kind of "self-medication" to relieve unpleasant emotions. In obesity, similar patterns of abuse using eating (seeking immediate gratification, using food to reduce unpleasant feelings) have been observed. Recently published studies have shown a surprisingly strong association between ADHD and obesity. In this study nearly half of patients with obesity had ADHD. The reasons for this strong association are unknown.

CANCER

Cancers known to be associated with overweight and obesity (a partial list):
Pancreatic cancer
Breast cancer
Uterine cancer
Cervical cancer
Kidney cancer
Bladder cancer
Esophageal cancer
Colon cancer
Stomach cancer
Liver cancer
Prostate cancer
Endometrial cancer
Multiple myeloma
Non-Hodgkin's lymphoma
Lung cancer
Melanoma

IN A LANDMARK STUDY ON OBESITY PUBLISHED IN THE *NEW ENGLAND Journal of Medicine* in 2003, nine hundred thousand U.S. adults were studied who were free of cancer at enrollment in 1982. The relationship in both men and women between BMI and the risk of death from all cancers was studied during a sixteen-year follow-up. The heaviest members of this cohort, with a BMI greater than 40, had death rates from all cancers that were 52 percent higher (men) and 62 percent higher (women) than the rates in men and women of normal weight. In both men and women, increased BMI was associated with higher rates of death from cancer of the esophagus, stomach, prostate, colon, rectum, liver, gallbladder, pancreas, kidney, breast, uterus, cervix, ovary, non-Hodgkin's lymphoma, and multiple myeloma. The positive association between certain cancers and increased BMI was of greater magnitude in those individuals who never smoked. Based on the associations observed in this study, the current patterns of overweight and obesity in the United States could account for 14 percent of all deaths of cancer in men and 20 percent of those in women. The public health implications for the United States are profound: more than ninety thousand deaths per year from cancer might be avoided if everyone in the adult population could maintain a BMI under 25 throughout life.

Pancreatic Cancer

Cancer of the pancreas represents the fifth leading cause of cancer-related mortality in the United States. Obesity has been shown to significantly increase the risk of pancreatic cancer in both men and women (the death rate is 40 to 50 percent higher for those with a BMI of 35 to 40). This finding may be explained by abnormal glucose intolerance and abnormally high insulin levels, as there is a strong association between diabetes and cancer of the pancreas. Studies have indicated a twofold increase in fatal pancreatic cancer among individuals with high blood sugar. The leading cause of type 2 diabetes is obesity.

Moderate exercise, defined as walking or hiking one and a half hours per week, is associated with a 50 percent reduction in pancreatic cancer risk in both men and women.

Breast Cancer

Breast cancer is the most common cancer in women (excluding skin cancer). Numerous studies of postmenopausal women have consistently revealed an increased breast cancer risk associated with obesity (a recent

New England Journal of Medicine article reported it was four times higher than for the nonobese), and a number of investigators have reported a decreased risk associated with physical activity. In addition, breast cancer patients who are obese are diagnosed later and have lower survival rates compared to nonobese breast cancer patients. Breast cancer risk can significantly be reduced with moderate to strenuous activity and weight loss—an amazing statement considering the number of lives that can be positively impacted.

Uterine Cancer

Uterine cancer is the fourth leading cause of cancer in women in the United States and is the most common female pelvic malignancy. Obesity has been found to be a consistent risk factor for uterine cancer. Women with a BMI of 35 to 40 have an increased risk of over one and a half times the nonobese of dying of this disease. A mechanism believed to increase the risk of uterine cancer is higher insulin levels, which occurs in the obese, as elevated insulin can increase the levels of sex hormones and growth factors that have a direct carcinogenic effect on uterine tissue. Because diabetes is positively associated with obesity, the apparent risk of uterine cancer in diabetic women may reflect this shared risk. The additional conferred risk of diabetes is apparent only in women with a BMI greater than 27.4. Diabetes alone does not increase risk of uterine cancer in normal-weight individuals.

Cervical Cancer

Overweight women with a BMI greater than 25 have a twofold increase in adenocarcinoma of the cervix compared to women who are not overweight. Fat tissue is not an inert substance; it can secrete its own hormones and can influence sex hormone levels. Fat tissue is known to convert the male sex hormones to estrogen, particularly in postmenopausal women. It is possible that this persistently elevated level of estrogen may be the mechanism that predisposes overweight women to an increased risk of cervical cancer.

Because of this higher incidence among obese women, I recommend that women who are overweight have a vaginal exam with a Pap smear at least once a year, and ideally twice a year.

Kidney Cancer

The incidence of kidney cancer in the United States is around thirty thousand cases, causing approximately twelve thousand deaths per year. Kidney cancer is the most rapidly increasing tumor type in the United States, which may be related to the rapid rise of obesity in our population. The strongest associations are with cigarette smoking, obesity, and hypertension.

Studies underscore the importance of even a small excess of body mass index and blood pressure in the development of kidney cancer and suggest that effective control of weight and blood pressure are useful in preventing this type of cancer. For obese individuals with a BMI of 35 to 40, their relative risk for kidney cancer is 70 percent greater than in individuals with a BMI of 25 or less. Investigators have shown an increase in kidney cancer among men consuming high-fat diets as well. Others point to an association between high consumption of fried meats and protein with chronic kidney diseases that may predispose to kidney cancer.

Bladder Cancer

Bladder cancer is the sixth most commonly diagnosed cancer in the United States. The *New England Journal of Medicine* recently reported an increased incidence of bladder cancer for those with a BMI greater than 30, with a relative risk of 34 percent higher for women and 14 percent for men compared to nonobese men and women. A longtime patient of mine in his fifties tragically died of bladder cancer a couple of years ago. His BMI was around 30, and he came in to see me because he'd had blood in his urine. His cancer had a rapid course and was incurable. I'll tell you the rest of the story not because it has anything to do with health, but because it touched me so deeply. His wife told me the story of how, when they were young newlyweds, a kind landlord had taken pity on them and let them rent a small room from him with no money down. When it came time for her husband to die so many years later, they took him to the hospice center at Beth Israel Hospital, built by a wealthy philanthropist. The wife said it was a beautiful, magnificent place that helped make his death a beautiful, moving experience. It turned out that their first landlord had gone on to make millions in public relations, and it was his name that went across the building. The wife's eyes welled up with tears when she told me how this wonderful man had taken care of them at a time when they needed him the most, both at the beginning of their married life together and the end.

Dietary factors also contribute to the development of bladder cancer. For example, high consumption of fried meats and fats increase the risk for bladder cancer. Fruit and vegetable intake, especially of cruciferous vegetables (such as broccoli, cauliflower, and brussels sprouts), has been found to be protective. Vitamin supplements, such as vitamin A, may also be protective.

Esophageal Cancer

Cancer of the esophagus is rare in the United States but extremely lethal. In the United States, most esophageal cancers are attributed to excess consumption of alcohol (especially whiskey) and long-term smoking. In addition, the association between BMI and esophageal cancer is strong in both men and women. For example, the relative risk for esophageal cancer in men who never smoked and who have a BMI between 35 and 40 is 91 percent greater compared to men with a BMI of 25 or less who never smoked. The carcinogenic mechanism is unknown.

Colon Cancer

Colon cancer is the second leading cause of cancer death in the United States, second only to lung cancer. Westernization or industrialization leads to an increased risk of colon cancer. A diet high in red meat or fat and low in fruits and vegetables increases the risk for this malignancy. Obesity, particularly abdominal adiposity, and physical inactivity are independent risk factors for colon cancer. Men with a BMI of 35 to 40 have an 84 percent increased risk of death from it, while for women it is 36 percent higher. The sedentary lifestyle may account in part for the higher rates of colon cancer in industrialized countries and urban areas. Numerous studies have pointed to an association between increased body mass and an elevated risk for colon cancer in men, although this association is weaker in women. This decreased risk in women compared to men may be related to the increased prevalence of central obesity in men.

Stomach Cancer

For unclear reasons, the incidence of stomach cancer has increased dramatically in the United States. The relative risk of stomach cancer steadily rises with increasing body mass, especially for men, who are at almost two times the risk of dying from it compared to normal-weight men. Nearly half of the cancers in the gastroesophageal region can be related to obesity and smoking. Though the strength and close dependency of the association between BMI and stomach cancer is striking, the mechanism that would fully explain this carcinogenic effect remains to be identified.

Liver Cancer

Liver cancer is one of the most common tumors in the world. Obesity is associated with an increased risk for cancer of the liver. Women with a BMI of 35 to 40 have a 68 percent higher death rate, while obese men have a four and a half times higher risk than normal-weight individuals. Cirrhosis is generally considered to be the most important risk factor for liver cancer, because almost all liver cancers are diagnosed after cirrhosis has developed, regardless of the original cause of liver damage. Obesity is also associated with an increased risk of cirrhosis, which may explain why the prevalence of liver cancer is increased in obesity.

Obese individuals will often develop what is called fatty liver disease as fat infiltrates the liver. Approximately 20 percent of our population has fatty liver disease. Fatty liver disease has slowly surpassed hepatitis C as the leading cause for hepatitis, which is a precursor for cirrhosis. In addition, more and more researchers have raised the intriguing possibility that obesity-related fatty liver itself is a pre-malignant condition.

Prostate Cancer

Cancer of the prostate is the most common malignancy in men in the United States and the third most common cause of cancer death in men above the age of fifty-five. A healthy diet appears to be a preventive measure in the development of prostate cancer. It has been reported that a reduced risk is associated with increased intake of fruits and vegetables. In another study, lycopene, an ingredient in tomatoes, was associated with a lower risk of prostate cancer. Numerous publications have also shown that a high-fat diet increases prostate cancer risk, although the mechanisms are not clear. In addition, it has been reported that animal fat may be the cause of a rise in prostate cancer, versus other fats such as vegetable or fish oils. High calorie intake in general may also be related.

There is no strong support for an association between BMI and prostate cancer. However, data do suggest a 20 to 34 percent increase of advanced prostate cancer or death among patients with a high BMI.

Endometrial Cancer

Cancer of the uterus is the most common female pelvic malignancy. Endometrial cancer, which originates in the inner lining of the uterus, accounts for about 90 percent of uterine cancers. Obesity is a known risk factor for endometrial cancer. The worldwide incidence of endometrial cancer correlates with estimates of per capita fat consumption. Women who are twenty to forty pounds above their ideal body weight have a threefold increase in risk, and women greater than forty pounds above their ideal body weight have a ninefold increase in risk of endometrial cancer when compared to matched controls of women at their ideal body weight. Inactivity and high calorie intake seem to be major risk factors of endometrial cancer independent of BMI. Furthermore, combined obesity and coexisting metabolic disturbances (increased blood pressure, increased blood sugar) may act synergistically to predispose to formation of cancer cells of the uterus.

Multiple Myeloma

Multiple myeloma is a malignancy of a type of immune system cell called a B cell. There is an elevated risk of multiple myeloma associated with being overweight and obese, with a stronger effect of BMI in women than in men. Men who have a BMI of 35 to 40 have a 71 percent higher death rate from it, while women in this range have a 44 percent higher risk. The mechanism linking high BMI to multiple myeloma is unclear, but some studies suggest that excess calorie intake and obesity may be involved in the development of this malignancy. The intake of fish, cruciferous vegetables, and vitamin supplements may decrease the risks. The increase of overweight and obesity in the United States over the last fifteen years may account for the 14 percent increase of multiple myeloma in the United States.

Non-Hodgkin's Lymphoma

Non-Hodgkin's lymphoma—cancers of lymphoid tissue (lymph nodes, spleen, and other organs of the immune system)—ranks as the sixth most common cause of cancer-related death in the United States. There is an association between overweight and obesity and non-Hodgkin's lymphoma; the relative risk for men in the highest BMI category is 50 percent and for women in the highest BMI category 95 percent, compared to nonobese age-matched individuals. Obesity also predisposes you to a higher risk of treatment failure and potential side effects.

Dietary factors also play a part in the risk. High intake of beef, pork, or lamb has been associated with an increased risk of non-Hodgkin's lymphoma. Higher consumption of vegetables, particularly cruciferous vegetables, and dietary fiber from vegetables was related to a lower risk.

Lung Cancer

As a lung specialist, I sadly see more lung cancer than most other doctors. It also happens to be one of the most preventable deadly diseases in medicine. Unfortunately, by the time the diagnosis is made the cancer often has already spread to the point that many patients are not surgical candidates for cure. In my opinion it is one of the worst types of deaths that a doctor has to see a patient through.

Lung cancer is the leading cause of cancer death of both men and women in the United States. While smoking is the most important risk factor, high BMI is also a risk factor. Those with a BMI greater than 30 have two times the incidence compared to those who have a BMI of 21. If you are obese *and* smoke, your chances of developing lung cancer are much higher compared to those who are of normal weight and don't smoke. Therefore, if you smoke or are a former smoker and have a BMI greater than 30, I recommend that you lose weight, stop smoking, and get a screening CAT scan of the lungs every year. Screening chest X-rays done on routine yearly physical exams are sometimes not sensitive enough to pick up early cases of lung cancer.

Melanoma

Malignant melanoma has been one of the most rapidly increasing cancers within the United States, with few modifiable risk factors outside of early sunburn prevention. It is a cancer that originates from the pigment cells of our skin. Its incidence has increased dramatically—300 percent in the last forty years.

Although I have not found a significant association between BMI and melanoma, I did find an association between melanoma and diet. Studies suggest that certain nutrients may protect against development of this cancer. Carotenoids (alpha-carotene, beta-carotene, cryptoxanthin, lutein, and lycopene, found in many fruits and vegetables), vitamin D, and retinol are associated with a decreased risk for melanoma. The protective effect of carotenoids for melanoma has been seen at levels easily obtained from the Mediterranean Prescription. No additional benefit is obtained through the use of supplements.

DECREASED IMMUNE FUNCTION

THE NORMAL FUNCTION OF THE IMMUNE SYSTEM IS ESSENTIAL FOR HEALTH. Dysfunction of the immune system can lead to a wide variety of diseases. Deficiency of immune-cell production or defective immune-cell function can lead to a spectrum of immunodeficiency diseases. On the other hand, overactivity of several of its components can lead to the development of allergic or autoimmune diseases. Leukemias and lymphomas are cancers that result from the malignant transformation of these cells.

Obesity has been related to immune dysfunction, which is accompanied by a higher rate of infection and increased risk of delayed wound healing. More importantly, a study published in 1980 demonstrated that 38 percent of obese children and adolescents showed a variable impairment of cell-mediated immunity (an important line of the body's defense, which gives us the capability of killing foreign cells or virus-infected cells). This affects how the body responds to vaccinations; simply explained, if your child is obese, he or she is less likely to be protected by the vaccinations he or she receives. Other researchers have since suggested that blood cholesterol, triglycerides, and glucose levels may be related to impairments in several aspects of immunity, although BMI has emerged as the most important factor. Ineffective antibody responses to vaccination in overweight adults has also been documented.

GALLBLADDER DISEASE

Gallbladder disease accounts for a considerable proportion of all hospitalizations related to digestive diseases in the United States. The gallbladder is a small sac that sits below the liver in the right upper abdomen just below the right diaphragm. The purpose of the gallbladder is to store and secrete bile into the small intestine in response to the ingestion of fats and amino acids. Bile is a solution of water, salts, lecithin, cholesterol, and other substances; if the concentration of these components changes, they may precipitate from solution and form gallstones. Gallstones are very prevalent in the United States. In one autopsy series, gallstones were shown to be present in 20 percent of women and men over the age of forty.

There are several important mechanisms in the formation of gallstones. The most important is increased cholesterol in the bile fluid. This may occur in association with obesity, pregnancy, very-low-calorie diets, high-calorie diets, or drugs. Approximately 10 to 25 percent of people losing weight rapidly through very-low-calorie dieting develop gallstones. Additionally, 35 to 38 percent of patients with morbid obesity develop gallstones as they lose weight after bariatric surgery.

It is well known that women with increased body size and central adiposity and who are on hormone replacement therapy are at significant increased risk. If these three factors can be modified, the incidence of gallbladder disease can be markedly reduced in women. In men and women, it is now suspected that high insulin levels and a poor lipid profile are independent risk factors for gallbladder disease. If these two factors can be modified, again, the incidence of gallbladder disease can be reduced. In addition, a relation between gallbladder disease and coronary heart disease has been reported, and it has been hypothesized that the two diseases may share a common etiology in hyperinsulinemia (high insulin).

GOUT

Gout is the deposition of uric acid crystals in any joint of the body. The disorder causes painful arthritis, especially in the joints of the feet and legs. Classically, gout is thought to be a disease of men, which begins with a sudden onset and involves a single joint, usually in the lower extremities.

Several factors may influence the development of gout, and study after study identifies obesity as one of the major modifiable risk factors. The coexistence of increased uric acid levels and cardiovascular disease is well established. Increased uric acid levels not only portend the possibility of heart disease but also represent a considerably increased risk for reduced life expectancy from other causes: in increasing order, the relative risk of death from all causes, coronary heart disease, stroke, liver disease, and kidney failure. These associations are so strong that any modifiable risk should be addressed. This includes weight loss, decreasing blood pressure, and decreasing cholesterol.

Low intakes of fiber, folate, and vitamin C increase the risk of gout, along with decreased consumption of fruits and vegetables. Dietary recommendations that address the risks would include eating a low-calorie diet with 40 percent of calories derived from carbohydrates, 30 percent from protein, and 30 percent from fat, which the Mediterranean Prescription provides. Of course, the Mediterranean Prescription also offers an abundance of fruit and vegetables, which are rich in micronutrients including folate, vitamin C, and dietary fiber.

THE LIVER

Disorders of the liver affected by overweight and obesity:
Non-alcoholic fatty liver disease (NAFLD)
Non-alcoholic steatohepatitis (NASH)
Cirrhosis
Liver cancer

Non-Alcoholic Fatty Liver Disease (NAFLD)

Non-alcoholic fatty liver disease (NAFLD) is simply the infiltration of fat within the architecture of the liver, which causes it to enlarge. The prevalence of NAFLD averages approximately 20 percent, making this condition the most common liver disease in the United States. The most common risk factors associated with NAFLD include obesity, type 2 diabetes, and hyperlipidemia (increased fat in the blood). Simple fatty infiltration of the liver occurs in 70 percent of overweight patients who are 10 percent above ideal body weight and in nearly 100 percent of those who are morbidly obese (with a BMI greater than 40). Some modalities of therapy include the aggressive management of associated conditions, such as treatment of high triglycerides and cholesterol with lipid-lowering drugs, and the treatment of diabetes with the appropriate medications, but the simplest and best treatment would be to lose weight.

Non-Alcoholic Steatohepatitis (NASH)

In lay terms, non-alcoholic steatohepatitis (NASH) is merely inflammation of the liver (hepatitis) caused by fat infiltrating the liver. It is the progression of NAFLD to the point where liver cells are destroyed by the inflammation fat causes. Within a period of ten years, almost 20 percent of patients with NASH will progress to cirrhosis. Once cirrhosis develops, the only therapy available is liver transplant. The natural history of NASH can be divided into four phases: (1) development of fatty liver, (2) inflammation of liver cells, (3) death of liver cells, and (4) scarring of liver (fibrosis/cirrhosis).

One of the most significant risk factors for this form of hepatitis is obesity. In an autopsy study, fatty hepatitis was found in 18.5 percent of the markedly obese versus 2.7 percent of lean subjects. No therapy for NASH has been proven to be effective. Treatment should be focused on prevention, correcting the risk factors for NASH. Similar to the approach one should take in preventing NAFLD, one's strategy should be weight loss, an exercise program, treating diabetes, and treating the liver disorder. Fatty liver disease has replaced hepatitis C as the leading cause of hepatitis in the United States and therefore is now the leading cause of cirrhosis and liver cancer.

Cirrhosis

Cirrhosis is the medical term that defines the end stage of chronic liver scarring. Patients may suffer from many complications, including accumulation of fluid in the abdomen, bleeding disorders, increased pressure in certain abdominal blood vessels, and confusion or a change in the level of consciousness. It is an irreversible process for which little treatment is available. Therapy for cirrhosis and the care of patients usually revolves around treating its complications. Without a liver transplant, this is a fatal disease and one of the most difficult and challenging medical illnesses for a doctor. Cirrhosis is also one of the leading causes of liver cancer; if you have cirrhosis, your chances of developing liver cancer increase 3 percent every year.

Liver Cancer

The only treatment for liver cancer is surgical resection (removing part of the liver), as it offers the only chance for cure. Unfortunately, few patients have a resectable tumor at the time the diagnosis is made. As a result, survival is usually only one to two years after the diagnosis is made. This topic is discussed more thoroughly on page 245.

THE LUNGS

Disorders of the lungs affected by overweight and obesity:
Sleep apnea
Obesity hypoventilation syndrome
Asthma
Pulmonary embolism

Sleep Apnea

Sleep apnea is defined as the periodic cessation of the flow of air through the nose and mouth during sleep—a period of time when the person is not breathing, essentially suffocating because air cannot get into the lungs. In most patients, the duration of the breathing cessation is twenty to thirty seconds; in some patients it could be as long as two to three minutes. The pauses usually occur ten to fifteen times per hour. The episodes of airway obstruction cause fragmented sleep, which gives rise to neuropsychiatric and behavioral disturbances. Sleep apnea is one of the leading causes of daytime sleepiness, which encroaches on all daily activities, particularly reading, watching television, or driving. Several studies have demonstrated that motor vehicle accidents and job-related accidents occur two to three times more frequently in patients with sleep apnea compared to other patients.

Obesity is a major cause of sleep apnea, as it causes obstruction of the pharynx (the cavity between the mouth and the esophagus) with fatty deposition within the soft tissue of the pharynx or by compressing the pharynx with fat tissue in the neck. Significant predictors of the frequency and severity of sleep apnea are excess body weight, central obesity (apple-shaped body type), snoring, heart disease, diabetes, age (it's more prevalent in people older than sixty-five), pregnancy, male gender (men are at two to three times greater risk), and alcohol use. The typical patient I encounter in my practice is one who presents complaining of morning headache, daytime sleepiness, and fatigue, who has high blood pressure, who is obese, and whose spouse complains of the partner's snoring. The patient may actually fall asleep while talking to me! Another complaint is erectile dysfunction.

In addition to forced ventilation through the nose at night, weight loss appears to be one of the most effective means of reducing sleep apnea in overweight people. I notice a dramatic difference in my patients when they return to my office as they start losing weight. They have lived for many years with the above symptoms and thought that it was normal for them to feel that way, but once they begin to drop the weight they have much more energy.

Obesity Hypoventilation Syndrome

Obesity hypoventilation syndrome is a condition related to (but which can occur separately from) obstructive sleep apnea, in which an obese person does not breathe a sufficient amount of oxygen during sleep or while awake. It is generally a condition that afflicts the morbidly obese (BMI greater than 40). Patients will usually present with unexplained heart and lung failure (cardiorespiratory failure), excessive sleepiness, sleep-disordered breathing, and edema (usually swelling of the legs and feet). Sometimes patients have said to me that as their weight increased they noted that they just couldn't think straight. Decreased cognitive function related to obesity has been described in the medical literature and is easily reversible once weight loss occurs. Their typical complaints are also shortness of breath with minimal exertion, shortness of breath at night when lying down (which is improved when sitting up in bed), difficulty putting on their shoes, and daytime sleepiness. These symptoms are the result of breathing at a low lung volume, resulting from the added weight on the rib cage and abdomen. If this effect of weight is not corrected, with time physiologic changes occur that will cause the blood carbon dioxide to rise, the oxygen to decrease, and the heart to fail. Once these changes occur, the process becomes irreversible and the patient will have progressive shortness of breath from cardiorespiratory failure.

The simple therapy for this condition is weight loss. Other therapies include forced ventilation through the nose at night, supplemental oxygen, and at times surgery to decrease the oral obstruction to airflow if it exists.

Asthma

Asthma is a disease of the lungs that is characterized by irritability of the windpipes. It is manifested by a narrowing of the air passages, making it difficult to get air in and out of the lungs, giving rise to shortness of breath, coughing, and wheezing. In my experience as a lung specialist, there is no more distressing symptom than not being able to catch your breath.

The prevalence of both obesity and asthma has increased dramatically in recent decades. This parallel increase has raised the speculation that the two are causally related. Prospective studies support this possibility. Although the exact mechanism of how this occurs is not known, what is known for certain is that weight loss among obese patients with asthma results in improvements in clinical measures and quality of life. In my own practice, obese asthmatic patients who lose weight will require fewer medications to keep their asthma under control. This has the effect of decreasing costs and decreasing medication side effects.

In my experience in the intensive care unit, where the critically ill are admitted, approximately 50 percent of all patients who are there on any given day have a history of smoking, are obese, or are alcohol abusers. The illnesses arising from these conditions and practices are self-inflicted and for the most part avoidable.

Pulmonary Embolism

There are only a few medical reasons for death to occur suddenly: cardiac arrest, stroke, acute bleeding, and pulmonary embolism. Pulmonary embolism (a clot that travels to the lungs) is one of the leading causes of undiagnosed hospital deaths, accounting for 5 to 10 percent of all deaths that occur to patients while they are in the hospital. It is disheartening to see many patients who after successful surgery succumb to this fatal disease, which is all too common and increasing in frequency. There are many factors that can predispose patients to pulmonary embolism, one of which is obesity.

Eighty to 90 percent of all pulmonary emboli originate from blood clots in the lower extremities (legs), and when these clots break off they travel to the right side of the heart and get caught in the lungs. Published data continue to suggest that a BMI of greater than 30 is a risk factor for sudden death from acute pulmonary embolism. Since obesity is common in developed countries and the prevalence of morbid obesity is increasing, synergy with other risk factors has become evident (such as use of birth control pills), which may account for a greater number of deaths occurring from pulmonary embolism than previously calculated. Women who have a BMI greater than 30 should be cautioned not to use oral contraceptives or should lose weight before starting them, as their risk for lower-extremity blood clots and pulmonary embolism can be synergistically increased.

MATERNAL OBESITY AND PREGNANCY OUTCOMES

Increased risks to mother and child associated with overweight and obesity:
Elevated blood pressure
Preeclampsia
Gestational diabetes
Increased incidence of cesarean section
Infections
Phlebitis and pulmonary embolism
Respiratory complications
Birth defects
Increased fetal mortality and preterm delivery
Macrosomia (larger for gestational-age baby)
Miscarriage

Chronically Elevated Blood Pressure

Throughout this book I have listed the many complications of hypertension (see page 235). Elevated blood pressure, even if only slightly raised, is of particular danger to both mother and child during pregnancy. Elevated blood pressure can lead to a condition called preeclampsia.

Preeclampsia

There is nothing in medicine that is more frightening and devastating to a physician than the potential loss of a mother and unborn child. Preeclampsia and eclampsia are conditions that a pregnant woman predisposes herself to if she is obese. Preeclampsia usually occurs in the third trimester of first-time pregnant women. This syndrome includes hypertension, spilling of protein in the urine, fluid retention, bleeding disorder, salt retention, and hyperresponsive reflexes. Eclampsia occurs when preeclampsia is not controlled and progresses to convulsions.

It is clear that pregnant obese women with preexisting chronic hypertension are at three to ten times higher risk than normal-weight pregnant women. This is not unexpected, because obesity is a well-known risk factor for hypertension. Obese pregnant women have a two- to fourfold increase in the incidence of preeclampsia even after controlling for preexisting chronic hypertension. The risk of preeclampsia typically doubles with each 5- to 7-point increase in BMI. One way to potentially prevent the loss of life of both mother and fetus is simply to be of normal weight.

Gestational Diabetes

The incidence of gestational diabetes increases by ten times in obese women compared to normal-weight women. The effects of gestational diabetes on the mother are the same as the effects of high blood sugar in the non-pregnant woman (see page 263). They include metabolic syndrome, increased incidence of infection, need for medications such as insulin, electrolyte abnormalities, fatigue, and dehydration. All of these obviously pose a danger to both mother and fetus. Other complications of gestational diabetes are macrosomia (giving birth to a baby larger than gestational age) and birth defects (discussed below).

Increased Incidence of Cesarean Section

Many studies have reported an increased cesarean section rate in obese women due to multiple causes (failure to induce labor, fetal distress, abnormal presentation, and labor abnormalities), with cesarean rates in obese women as high as 30 percent.

Infections

Postoperative wound infection, infections of the uterus, and urinary tract infections are all associated with obesity. Because of this, it is now medically accepted practice to use prophylactic antibiotics during cesarean section in obese women to prevent postoperative infections.

Phlebitis and Pulmonary Embolism

Because pregnancy decreases blood flow from the veins of the lower extremities and pregnancy activates the clotting system, pregnant women are at higher risk for forming blood clots, particularly in the legs. These clots can break away and travel to the lungs, resulting in pulmonary embolism, a life-threatening condition. Obesity further increases this risk, especially if the obese pregnant woman undergoes a cesarean section. As a result of the increased risk, it has become accepted medical practice to place such patients on medications that thin the blood. Unfortunately, such drugs predispose obese pregnant women to the added risk of bleeding complications.

Respiratory Complications

Review of the literature demonstrates that obese children and nonpregnant adults are predisposed to an increased rate of asthma (see page 254) and sleep apnea (see page 252). Obese pregnant women are affected in a similar way: breathing takes more effort, their chest wall elasticity (ability to expand) decreases, and they have increased resistance of the air passages that makes it more difficult for the air to enter the lungs. All of the above factors are also components of asthma. The fetus is subsequently affected, as oxygen decreases during asthma attacks. Physicians often need to prescribe medications to treat these asthma attacks, again predisposing mother and fetus to possible adverse drug effects.

Obesity has been shown to be one of the major causes of sleep apnea. Sleep apnea is characterized by frequent episodes of not breathing while asleep, causing a decreased oxygen supply to the fetus. Although studies have not been done to determine if there is an adverse impact on pregnancy outcome, it cannot be beneficial to mother or fetus.

Birth Defects

Congenital Heart Defects

Heart defects affect at least 1 in 150 newborns and are among the most frequent major congenital abnormalities, contributing to excess complications, premature death, and health care costs. Recent findings suggest that there may be a relation between maternal BMI and the likelihood of having a child with a heart defect. Whatever mechanism is involved between pre-pregnancy weight and heart defects in offspring, it is likely to occur early in pregnancy. The heart forms early in the fetus; it is the first organ to function, beginning to pump during the fourth week of gestation. The four-chambered heart is basically formed by the eighth week of gestation, but some heart development continues beyond that period, allowing for additional malformations to occur.

Neural Tube Defects

Neural tube defects (NTDs) are congenital abnormalities resulting in malformations of the brain and/or spinal cord (anencephaly, spina bifida, craniorachischisis, or iniencephaly). Diabetes, pre-pregnancy obesity, increased insulin levels, and increased intake of sugars (sucrose, fructose, glucose) are all associated with an increased risk of NTDs. The interdependence of these factors suggests a common pathway via altered sugar control and insulin demand. An increased intake of sugars quadrupled the risk of NTDs in non-diabetic obese patients in a recent study. Other maternal nutritional factors have also been implicated in the cause of NTDs. The most important among these factors is folic acid intake early after conception. Additional factors such as increased intake of methionine, zinc, vitamin C, and dairy products have been shown to decrease the risk of NTDs. A well-balanced diet such as the Mediterranean Prescription provides much of this.

Increased Fetal Mortality and Preterm Delivery

Weight before pregnancy matters more than people realize, and overweight translates to an increased risk of fetal death. Obese pregnant women have an increased risk of delivering a premature baby before the thirty-second week of gestation. This is associated with a higher rate of fetal mortality. The risk of premature delivery in obese women is 5 to 7 per

1,000 deliveries. The studies that reported these findings corrected for diabetes and hypertension, which in my opinion underestimates the number of premature deliveries and fetal death.

Macrosomia

The term *macrosomia* is used to describe a newborn with a birth weight over a certain figure (8 pounds 13 ounces to 9 pounds 15 ounces, depending on gestational age, the sex of the fetus, and ethnicity). Factors that are associated with fetal macrosomia are diabetes during pregnancy, duration of pregnancy, maternal obesity and excessive maternal weight gain, and genetics. Macrosomia has been associated with newborn complications and disease, newborn injury, maternal injury, and cesarean delivery. When fetal macrosomia is associated with diabetes, it usually indicates poor sugar control in the mother, and these infants are at increased risk for stillbirth. Stillbirth rates in macrosomic infants are twice as high as those in control subjects irrespective of diabetes. A higher fetal mortality rate occurs with a birth weight of greater than 9 pounds 15 ounces in non-diabetic mothers and a birth weight of greater than 8 pounds 13 ounces in diabetic mothers.

Miscarriage

Miscarriage (spontaneous abortion) is a major complication in pregnancy and can occur in pregnancies from both natural conception and fertility treatment. Recurrent spontaneous abortion has been associated with obesity in the general population. To help increase the chances of keeping a pregnancy, maintaining optimal weight is the one thing that pregnant women have direct control over.

MUSCLES, BONES, AND CARTILAGE

Disorders of muscle, bone, and cartilage affected by overweight and obesity:
Carpal tunnel syndrome
Osteoarthritis of the knee
Osteoarthritis of the hip
Musculoskeletal pain
Rheumatoid arthritis
Chronic low back pain

Carpal Tunnel Syndrome

Carpal tunnel syndrome is the most common form of nerve damage observed in the general population. It is a condition caused by impingement of a nerve that passes through the wrist. The most typical symptoms are pain and a sensation of pins and needles in the hands. Other symptoms include lack of sensation in the hands, feeling pins and needles in the hands while reading or driving, and dropping objects; temporary relief of symptoms can be obtained by shaking the hands. Risk factors for developing carpal tunnel syndrome include obesity, female gender, age above thirty years, repetitive activity, diabetes, rheumatoid arthritis, hypothyroidism (underactive thyroid), smoking, and repetitive vibration. Most people assume that most cases are related to repetitive motion, but that's not true. Features of the workplace, other than vibration, are actually weak predictors of this disorder, and the other risk factors are stronger. Numerous studies have consistently shown that obesity/overweight (BMI greater than 27) is an independent risk factor for carpal tunnel syndrome. One study found an increased risk of 8 percent for each one-unit increase in BMI.

Osteoarthritis of the Knee

Osteoarthritis of the knee is the most prevalent chronic joint condition and the leading cause of disability in the United States. Osteoarthritis in general is the most common form of chronic arthritis and results in more functional loss than any other disease, including heart disease and cancer. It is quite strongly related to obesity. Obesity is also known to exacerbate pain and disability once the disease manifests with symptoms. Unfortunately, it is a disease that many of us are all too familiar with, seeing it in older friends and relatives suffering from limited mobility, limping, and knee pain. It is most commonly seen in older women, and it is a major cause of physical disability with aging, leading to loss of independence in the elderly.

The degree of obesity at an early age also affects the risk of developing knee osteoarthritis later in life. The most common symptoms of osteoarthritis are pain and stiffness. Because there is no known cure for this disease, except for knee replacement, the focus should be on prevention. Although osteoarthritis is a multifactorial disease with both genetic and environmental determinants, the risk of this disease could be significantly reduced with simple weight loss. A study published in 1992 revealed that a weight loss of approximately ten pounds over a ten-year period decreased the odds of developing significant knee osteoarthritis by more than 50 percent. Another study demonstrated that a 5 percent weight loss produced a statistically significant reduction in knee pain in obese women.

Osteoarthritis of the Hip

Osteoarthritis of the hip causes substantial disease and disability in the elderly, and it is the leading reason for hip replacements in the United States. There is no curative therapy for it except for hip replacement. Available treatment reduces symptoms and improves function but does not alter the disease process. Once structural damage to the joint cartilage occurs, causing joint space narrowing and bony overgrowth, the process cannot be reversed by standard therapeutic modalities. Risk factors for osteoarthritis include those that are fixed (e.g., age, sex, family history, and possibly race) as well as those that are amenable to modification (e.g., obesity, physical activity, exercise levels, muscle weakness, and joint injury). In the Nurses Health Study, which studied 120,000 women, it was found that higher BMI and age were the only risk factors for osteoarthritis of the hip requiring hip replacement. The risk estimates for higher BMI at age eighteen were significantly greater for development of hip osteoarthritis than those for the high BMIs reported closer to the date of surgery. This data suggests the importance of interventions to reduce obesity, particularly at younger ages. It has been estimated that if obesity were eliminated, the prevalence of hip osteoarthritis would decrease by 25 percent.

Musculoskeletal Pain

In a recently published study, it was shown that obese individuals face an increased risk of musculoskeletal pain and osteoarthritis. Obese people overload their knee and hip joints, which probably explains most of the increased risk of developing osteoarthritis. Mental distress also increases the risk of musculoskeletal pain. Work-restricting pain in the hip, knee, and ankle joints is more responsive to weight loss than pain in the neck and back areas, indicating that pain in joints is related to osteoarthritis and mechanical overload. The simple fact is that if obese people with hip, knee, or other joint pain were to lose weight, it is likely that some or all of their pain and achiness would go away.

Rheumatoid Arthritis

Rheumatoid arthritis is a chronic inflammatory disease of the joints that may have a variety of systemic manifestations. Family studies indicate a genetic predisposition. The cause of rheumatoid arthritis remains largely unknown, although microbiological, immune, genetic, hormonal, and dietary factors have been implicated.

Obesity has been found to be related to rheumatoid arthritis in both men and women. In addition, there are numerous studies pointing to dietary factors that can decrease this incidence. Specifically, dietary factors have been shown to affect experimentally induced polyarthritis in rats. Additionally, accumulating evidence from intervention studies in humans suggest that supplementation of the diet with fish oil or olive oil improves the symptoms of rheumatoid arthritis by altering the production of mediators of immunity and inflammation.

Chronic Low Back Pain

Changes in body composition are known to occur as we age. In particular, a decrease in lean body mass and an increase in fat are characteristic of the aging process. The consequences of these changes in lean body mass may include decreased muscle mass and muscle strength. A recent study reported that a high waist-to-hip ratio, indicating a central distribution of fat, was significantly associated with chronic low back pain in women (but not in men). Recently two population surveys have reported positive relationships between BMI and back pain, meaning that as weight increases, so does back pain. As pain increases, unfortunately, it creates a vicious circle; the less exercise we do, the more sedentary we become and the more weight we gain. This highlights the importance of prevention and early action, including weight loss.

THE PANCREAS

Disorders of the pancreas affected by overweight and obesity:
Pancreatitis
Pancreatic cancer
Type 2 diabetes
Diabetes and childhood obesity
The metabolic syndrome

Pancreatitis

The pancreas is the organ that produces insulin and digestive enzymes and is located behind the stomach. A condition called pancreatitis develops when it becomes inflamed. Pancreatitis can be extremely serious, with a mortality rate of 10 percent. Obese patients with acute pancreatitis tend to show increased complications and fatal outcomes. The risk of infectious complication such as abscesses, infected dead tissue, and infection of pancreatic origin is greater in obese patients. If the acute pancreatitis is related to alcohol use or gallstones, obesity is associated with an even higher risk for complications and a fatal outcome.

Pancreatic Cancer

See page 241.

Type 2 Diabetes

Type 2 diabetes is the most common form of diabetes. In type 2 diabetes, either the body does not produce enough insulin or the cells ignore the insulin. Insulin is necessary for the cells of our body to be able to use sugar. Sugar is the basic fuel for the cells in the body, and insulin takes the sugar from the blood into the cells. When glucose builds up in the blood instead of going into cells, it can cause two problems: cells will be starved for energy, and over time high blood glucose levels may damage the eyes, kidneys, nerves, and/or heart.

Type 2 diabetes is the most common hormonal disease worldwide and is characterized by metabolic abnormalities that affect almost every organ of our body. Type 2 diabetes is increasing in incidence worldwide primarily because of increases in the prevalence of a sedentary lifestyle and overweight and obesity. Physical activity and BMI are the main non-genetic determinants of this disease. Acute symptoms of diabetes vary from patient to patient and are usually related to the high blood sugar itself: frequent urination, excessive thirst, and excessive hunger. Less commonly, the first event may be an acute metabolic decompensation resulting in diabetic coma.

Prevention includes a combination of several lifestyle factors, including maintaining a BMI of 25 or lower, eating a diet high in fiber and unsaturated fat and low in saturated and trans fats, exercising regularly, abstaining from smoking, and consuming alcohol moderately, all of which are recommended in the Mediterranean Prescription. These measures are associated with a 90 percent lower risk of type 2 diabetes in women, a staggering finding.

In my office practice I rarely see a patient who requires heart surgery, has peripheral vascular disease, or has had a stroke who doesn't have diabetes or glucose intolerance. The reason for this has been clarified by recent studies that have transformed our thinking about fat cells, which are no longer regarded as passive depots that store energy but as active regulators of the pathways responsible for energy balance, controlled by a complex network of hormones and nerve signals. Fat cells secrete numerous substances that have an effect on insulin and the numerous vessels, arteries, veins, and capillaries in our body.

Diabetes and Childhood Obesity

The incidence of type 2 diabetes in childhood has skyrocketed in recent years, and while genes have a role in diabetes (close relatives of people with diabetes have a greater chance to develop it themselves), research has shown that diabetes is not caused by genetics alone. Other risk factors for type 2 diabetes include being overweight, physical inactivity, or belonging to certain ethnic groups (African American, Latino, Native American, and Asian Americans are at higher risk). While there are factors outside our control, some risk factors are modifiable. Certain lifestyle changes have been shown to reduce the severity of the condition or eliminate it altogether, the most important of these being keeping a healthy weight and keeping active.

The Metabolic Syndrome

One of the metabolic abnormalities that is associated with overweight and obesity is the metabolic syndrome (also called insulin resistance syndrome), which is diagnosed when three or more of the following conditions are present: increased weight around the abdomen, resistance to the effects of insulin, increased insulin levels, increased blood pressure, increased triglycerides and cholesterol, and increased sugar in the blood. Most of these conditions are exacerbated—if not caused—by excess weight. Dietary factors that have been linked to the metabolic syndrome are the ratios of monounsaturated or polyunsaturated to saturated fats ingested, dietary fiber, and consumption of sugar.

THE SKIN

Skin changes seen with overweight and obesity:
Acanthosis nigricans and skin tags
Hirsutism, baldness, and acne in women
Stretch marks
Varicose veins and stasis pigmentation
Lymphedema
Intertrigo
Cellulite
Callus formation
Pressure ulcers
Slow wound healing

Overweight and obesity can have numerous complications that affect the skin. Dermatological manifestations of obesity can range from annoying to incapacitating. Early recognition and treatment of these skin disorders and their complications is essential for appropriate care.

Acanthosis Nigricans and Skin Tags

Acanthosis nigricans is an eruption of brown, velvety, warty growths occurring on the skin in areas where the skin typically folds: the underarms, neck, anus and genital area, and groin. Skin tags are pinhead to grape-size flesh-colored polyps. They are seen most often on the eyelids, neck, and armpits. Skin tags can be unsightly and may become painful if the stem twists.

Both conditions commonly occur in obese individuals and have been observed in up to 74 percent of those who are obese. Their prevalence is correlated with the severity of obesity. Both are also associated with insulin resistance and increased circulating insulin levels (which are often found in the overweight and obese).

Hirsutism, Baldness, and Acne in Women

Obesity can cause hyperandrogynism, meaning the increased secretion of male hormones, in women. Fat tissue synthesizes testosterone. In obese women this can result in menstrual irregularities, hirsutism (male distribution of hair), male-pattern baldness, and acne. All of these conditions will resolve as insulin levels and insulin resistance decrease. This can be accomplished with medications that treat diabetes and by simply losing weight. The use of oral contraceptives has also been found to be effective.

Stretch Marks

Stretch marks (striae distensae) are linear, smooth bands of shriveled-appearing skin that at first appear reddish, then purple, and finally white, when they become depressed into the skin. These are common skin findings in obesity. They generally follow skin-fold lines and occur most commonly on the abdomen, buttocks, and groin regions. Treatment has been unsatisfactory once they are well formed. Effective treatment of stretch marks must be instituted during the active stage of formation, before the scarring process is complete.

Varicose Veins and Stasis Pigmentation

Some studies have found a significant association between obesity, varicose veins, and stasis pigmentation. Varicose veins are the unsightly, swollen veins on the surface that occur in the lower extremities and result from inadequate return of blood from the lower extremities. Stasis pigmentation is commonly seen in both lower extremities below the knees as small rust- or red-colored dots. Stasis pigmentation is usually the result of varicose veins because of the slow return of blood—blood cells die, and the pigmentation is the result of the iron carried by those blood cells being deposited under the skin.

The resulting inflammation and swelling may predispose patients to skin erosions, skin ulcers, and itching. Weight loss is the obvious treatment, along with the use of elastic stockings and topical steroids to alleviate the itching.

Lymphedema

The definition of *lymphedema* is swelling as a result of obstruction of lymphatic vessels or lymph nodes and the accumulation of increased amounts of lymph fluid in the affected region. In the obese patient, lymphedema develops because of an abnormal accumulation of protein-rich lymphatic fluid that occurs when lymphatic return is impaired. The onset is gradual, resulting in swelling of the legs. The swelling is painless and the patient will report that the swelling disappears overnight. In late stages, the swelling becomes hardened and the skin thickens. Recurrent skin infections usually result. Treatment for this condition is directed at reducing limb girth, weight loss, and preventing infection.

Intertrigo

Intertrigo occurs when skin surfaces rub against each other and become irritated and inflamed. Excessive fat folds in patients with obesity lead to friction between skin surfaces and maceration of the skin from accumulated moisture in the folds, causing a scaling, reddish rash. Patients with obesity become overheated easily and sweat more profusely because of the thick layers of fat. Infection can occur with bacteria, fungus, or yeast. Common areas include the groin, under the breast, the armpit, the abdominal wall, and the buttocks. Patients may complain of itching or burning over the affected areas. Treatment for this condition includes weight loss, antifungal creams, antibiotics, and/or oral antifungal drugs.

Cellulite

Technically, cellulite is the deposits of fat and fibrous tissue that cause dimpling of the overlying skin. Cellulite is not exclusively related to obesity but is usually accentuated by it and is common particularly in women. Treatment, though not especially effective, includes exercise, dietary modification, and increased water intake.

Callus Formation

Callus formation on the feet (plantar hyperkeratosis) is the most common finding in patients with excessive obesity. This is caused by the abnormal transference of excess weight during the walking cycle. The use of insoles helps to alleviate symptoms while control of obesity is being achieved.

Pressure Ulcers

Pressure ulcers usually develop over bony prominences or within soft tissue exposed to prolonged and unrelieved pressure. However, patients who are obese may develop skin breakdown and ulceration in areas other than the tissue over bony prominences. This may result from capillary closure within folds of fat, which can create ulceration and tissue destruction.

Slow Wound Healing

Obesity impairs wound healing by decreasing blood flow to the affected skin. This decreases the delivery of oxygen and nutrients to the wound, which slows tissue repair and wound healing. Tension on the wound edges may further slow wound healing.

THE STOMACH

Disorders of the stomach affected by overweight and obesity:
Gastroesophageal reflux disease
Esophageal cancer
Stomach cancer

Gastroesophageal Reflux Disease

Gastroesophageal reflux disease (GERD) is a disease caused by reflux of stomach or intestinal contents into the esophagus, which causes damage to the lining of the esophagus. Reflux is more likely to occur when the stomach is full, after meals, when there is too much acid produced by the stomach, when lying down, in the presence of a hiatal hernia, or when stomach pressure is increased, such as with obesity, pregnancy, and wearing girdles. Medications can also cause reflux along with fatty foods, fried foods, chocolate, caffeine, and smoking.

Reflux symptoms and obesity are strong and independent risk factors for esophageal cancer, a cancer that has increased significantly in incidence during recent decades. There is a strong association between increasing BMI and reflux in women, and a moderate association among men. In a recent study, a reduction of BMI was associated with a significantly decreased incidence of reflux symptoms.

Esophageal Cancer

See page 244.

Stomach Cancer

See page 245.

SURGICAL INFECTIONS

SURGICAL SITE INFECTIONS ARE THE MOST COMMON INFECTIONS THAT occur in the hospital setting for those patients who are operated on. They contribute to increased complications, resulting in longer hospital stays and increased cost. There is an association between high BMI and surgical site infection. The increased incidence of this in the obese is due to an increase in local tissue trauma related to retraction, a lengthened operative time, and local changes that occur due to increased fat tissue. One study found that patients with surgical site infections were twice as likely to die, 60 percent more apt to be admitted to an intensive care unit postoperatively, and over five times more likely to require hospital readmission.

HERNIAS

OBESITY IS AMONG ONE OF THE RISK FACTORS THAT SEEMS TO BE STRONGLY predictive for hernia occurrence. In addition, there is a strong association between obesity and the recurrence of hernia (particularly of the groin area) after repair. As a result, such patients will frequently have a mesh rather than a suture repair, which in some studies has been found to have a higher rate of infectious complications.

UROLOGICAL DISEASE

Urological disorders affected by overweight and obesity:
Kidney disease*
Enlarged prostate*
Erectile dysfunction/impotence
Prostate cancer*
Kidney cancer*
Overactive bladder and stress urinary incontinence*
Varicocele (impaired drainage of testicular veins)

* Described below

Kidney Disease

Our kidneys are responsible for the vital job of regulating our body water. Five-year survival for people with end-stage kidney (renal) disease is less than 50 percent. Risk factors for the progression of kidney disease include hypertension, obesity, diabetes, hyperlipidemia, high-protein diet, and physical inactivity, all of which are modifiable by the diet and exercise program of the Mediterranean Prescription.

There are three mechanisms that appear to be important factors linking hypertension, obesity, and the kidneys: (1) secretion by fatty tissue of a hormone that stimulates the nervous system and leads to hypertension, causing injury to the kidneys; (2) activation of hormones (renin-angiotensin system) causing salt retention, again leading to hypertension and kidney injury; and (3) altered forces within the kidney due to the direct mass effect of fat, which causes decreased kidney function, resulting in hypertension and further kidney disease.

Enlarged Prostate

Enlarged prostate (benign prostatic hypertrophy) is a condition that is not a major cause of death but continues to be a leading cause of disease in elderly men. The prostate gland surrounds the urethra, and an enlarged prostate is the most common cause of obstruction to urinary outflow in men. This is a universal condition in aging men. By age twenty the prostate weighs about 20 grams, and it will remain stable in size for twenty-five years. In the fifth decade it starts to grow in the majority of men, and by the age of forty-five most men will suffer from this condition. When severe enough, the urine backs up into the kidneys and can cause kidney failure. In an article published in a urology journal in 1996, obesity was found to predispose men to this condition.

Prostate Cancer

See page 245.

Kidney Cancer

See page 243.

Overactive Bladder and Stress Urinary Incontinence

Several studies have assessed the association of urinary incontinence with lifestyle factors such as smoking, alcohol intake, and physical inactivity. Associations with obesity have also been made for those suffering with overactive bladder and stress incontinence. Increased consumption of chicken, vegetables, and bread was associated with reduced risk of overactive bladder and onset of stress incontinence.

Many men and women are reluctant to complain of these symptoms. They may feel embarrassed to discuss it. While performing a physical examination, the doctor can usually tell if a patient is suffering from stress incontinence by the aroma of urine (patients usually don't notice it because they're used to it) and the urine stains on their underwear. If the patient is obese, the recommendation is to lose weight.

WOMEN'S INFERTILITY

Thousands of years ago Hippocrates had already recognized the influence of obesity on reproductive function in his writings on infertility: "Fatness and flabbiness are to blame. The womb is unable to receive the semen and they menstruate infrequently." Fat tissue actually does play a significant role in the metabolism of sex hormones, causing decreased ovulation cycles or no ovulation at all in obese women, resulting in infertility. Obese women with a BMI greater than 27 have a threefold risk of failure-to-ovulate infertility compared with women with a BMI of 20 to 25.

Obese women have a multitude of hormonal abnormalities: insulin resistance, increased insulin levels, increased male hormones (androgens), increased conversion of male hormones to estrogens, decreased growth hormone, increased leptin levels, and altered regulation of the pituitary-ovary axis that regulates menstruation. As a result of the increase of some hormones and decrease of others, the ovulation cycle in obese women is altered, possibly explaining the relationship between obesity and infertility.

Polycystic Ovary Syndrome

Polycystic ovary syndrome (PCOS) is the most common endocrinological (hormonal) disorder in women of reproductive age, affecting about 6 percent of women. Obesity is present in around 50 percent of patients. Obesity contributes to the manifestations of PCOS and infertility by increasing testosterone levels and increasing the rates of failed ovulation cycles. This results from increased insulin levels, which we all now know is one of the most common results of obesity. There is therapy for this disorder that involves the use of a medicine called metformin, but obese women are less likely to respond. Obese women who lose weight are more likely to respond to this therapy and can possibly have normal ovarian function restored.

Appendix B

Vitamins, Phytochemicals, and Other Micronutrients: What They Do and Where to Find Them

Please note that the potential health benefits listed below are primarily related to consuming the listed vitamins and phytochemicals in their natural food sources, as I promote in the Mediterranean Prescription, not via supplements. Colorful fruits and vegetables contain hundreds and possibly thousands of phytochemicals that work together with nutrients to promote health and prevent disease. When you eat fruits and vegetables, the phytochemicals are easily absorbed and provide the maximum health benefits. In contrast, supplements or pills contain large doses of only one or two phytochemicals. Supplement studies have mostly been disappointing, showing ineffectiveness and in some cases even harm (for example, incidence of stroke increased with vitamin E supplementation, and at very high doses [> 2,000 IU/day] death from all causes increased).

MICRO-NUTRIENT	WHAT IT IS	POTENTIAL HEALTH BENEFITS	WHERE IT'S FOUND
Alpha-carotene (gets converted to vitamin A)	Member of the carotenoid family; antioxidant	• Anti-cancer (especially lung) • Necessary for normal growth as well as healing • Helps maintain eyesight • Helps maintain immune function	Carrots, sweet potatoes, apricots, pumpkins, cantaloupes, green beans, lima beans, broccoli, brussels sprouts, cabbage, kale, kiwi, lettuce, peas, spinach, prunes, peaches, mangoes, papayas, squash
Alpha-linolenic acid	Belongs to the group of omega-3 fatty acids	• Reduces inflammation • Lowers cholesterol • Anti-cancer (breast) • Improves immunity • Reduced risk of heart attack • Anti-obesity and thermogenic effects may be related to the stimulation of lipid metabolism in the small intestine • Helps neurological function, such as mitigating depression and stress	Flaxseed, flaxseed oil, walnuts, cold-water fish (such as salmon, mackerel, tuna, sardines, anchovies), green leafy vegetables (such as kale, broccoli, brussels sprouts), canola oil
Anthocyanins	Polyphenol subgroup of flavonoids; antioxidant	• Anti-cancer • Anti-inflammatory • Protects against heart-related diseases • Helps lower blood sugar • Protects against diabetes • Supports the nervous system • Benefits skin and collagen	Red wine, grapes, bilberries, blueberries, elderberries, cranberries, prunes, red cabbage, eggplant, apples
Arginine	An amino acid made naturally in the body	• May help prevent heart disease	Nuts, some dairy products, poultry, fish

MICRO-NUTRIENT	WHAT IT IS	POTENTIAL HEALTH BENEFITS	WHERE IT'S FOUND
Beta-carotene (gets converted to vitamin A)	Member of the carotenoid family; antioxidant	• Anti-cancer • May prevent cataracts • May slow progression of heart disease • Boosts immune system	Sweet potatoes, carrots, melons, pumpkins, mangoes, cantaloupes, papayas, peaches, prunes, squash, apricots, cabbage, lima beans, green beans, broccoli, brussels sprouts, kale, kiwi, lettuce, peas, spinach, tomatoes, pink grapefruit, honeydew melon, oranges
Carotenoids	Subgroup of polyphenols; fat-soluble; antioxidant	• Anti-cancer (especially breast and lung) • Reduces risk of cataracts • Reduces risk of coronary artery disease • Enhances immunity in the elderly	Some of the many foods that contain carotenoids are pineapples, citrus fruits, peaches, nectarines, persimmons, tomatoes, papayas, apricots, carrots, watermelons, pumpkins, squashes, sweet potatoes, spinach, broccoli, collard greens, kale
Catechins	Antioxidant flavonoid	• Anti-cancer • Protects against chemically induced cancers and skin cancer	Green and black tea, berries
Curcumin	Polyphenolic compound with antioxidant and anti-inflammatory properties; curcumin gives turmeric and curry its bright yellow color	• Anti-cancer • Reduces skin cancer risk • Has been found to reduce gastric, colon, bladder, and lung cancers in the laboratory • May lower cholesterol • May have protective effects upon Alzheimer's disease	Tumeric, curry powder, mustard (small amounts)

MICRO-NUTRIENT	WHAT IT IS	POTENTIAL HEALTH BENEFITS	WHERE IT'S FOUND
Flavonoids	Subgroup of polyphenols (phenolic compounds) comprising more than 4,000 types; give plants color, are antifungal, antioxidants	• Lower cholesterol • Anti-cancer • Prevent blood clotting • Anti-inflammatory • Anti-bacterial	Oranges, apples, grapefruits, onions, white cabbage, berries, juices, red wine, chocolate, tea
Folacin (folate/folic acid)	Water-soluble B vitamin that occurs naturally in food	• Helps produce and maintain new cells, which is especially important during periods of rapid cell division and growth such as infancy and pregnancy • May lower blood levels of homocysteine, which has been linked to cardiovascular disease • Anti-cancer (especially colon)	Beans, avocadoes, artichokes, asparagus, spinach, turnip greens, rice, peas, broccoli, peanuts, lettuce, wheat germ, beef liver, tomato and orange juices, fortified cereals
Glucosinolates	Produces the bioactive compound isothiocyanates (thorough chewing of the vegetable makes them available)	• Anti-cancer	Cruciferous vegetables such as broccoli, cauliflower, cabbage, brussels sprouts, kale, turnips, bok choy
Indoles	A group of phytochemicals; effects may increase with cooking	• Anti-cancer (may protect against hormone-related cancers such as those of the prostate and breast)	Cruciferous vegetables such as broccoli, cauliflower, cabbage, brussels sprouts, kale, turnips, bok choy
Isoflavones	Estrogen-like flavonoid	• Anti-cancer; possibly guard against hormone-related cancers such as breast cancer	Soybeans

MICRO-NUTRIENT	WHAT IT IS	POTENTIAL HEALTH BENEFITS	WHERE IT'S FOUND
Isothiocyanates	Sulfur-containing phytochemicals	• Anti-cancer; stimulate the body to break down carcinogens	Cruciferous vegetables such as broccoli, cauliflower, cabbage, brussels sprouts, kale, turnips, bok choy, radishes, mustard greens
Lutein	Fat-soluble, antioxidant carotenoid	• May help prevent macular degeneration, the leading cause of blindness in people over 65	Spinach, kale, collard greens, romaine lettuce, leeks, peas
Lycopene	Potent antioxidant	• Anti-cancer (especially breast and prostate) • May help protect skin from ultraviolet radiation • May reduce risk of cardiovascular disease	Tomatoes, tomato paste and sauce, ketchup, watermelon, red grapefruit, dried apricots
Organosulfides	Phytochemicals that give onions etc. their distinctive taste and smell; may degrade after cooking	• Anti-cancer (especially prostate) • Lowers cholesterol • Lowers blood pressure • Helps fight gut infections • Anti-blood-clotting agent in arteries	Allium vegetables such as onions, garlic, leeks, shallots, chives
Pectin	A soluble fiber that gels the cell walls of plants together	• Acts as appetite suppressant: fiber gel slows digestion so you feel full longer • Anti-cancer (colon) • Helps prevent heart disease • Lowers cholesterol • Helps diabetics control blood sugar levels • Aids digestion • Reduces atherosclerosis (hardening of the arteries) • Helps those suffering from ulcer or colitis • Helps regulate blood pressure • Effective in preventing gallstones	Peaches, apples, currants, plums, grapefruits, beets, oranges, cranberries, Concord grapes, quinces, gooseberries, crabapples

MICRO-NUTRIENT	WHAT IT IS	POTENTIAL HEALTH BENEFITS	WHERE IT'S FOUND
Polyphenols	Subgroup of phytochemicals; most abundant source of antioxidants in our diet	• Anti-cancer	Fruits (esp. apple, pear, grape), vegetables (esp. onion, red peppers, celery), wheat bran, soy, green and black tea, red wine, coffee, chocolate
Quercetin	Antioxidant flavonoid; apparently remains intact after cooking	• Anti-cancer • Associated with reduced risk of heart disease • Inhibits blood clotting	Wine, onions, tea
Selenium	Element found on the periodic table, a trace mineral; antioxidant that complements vitamin E in stimulating the immune system; must be present in the soil for the plant to contain it	• Anti-cancer • Protects against heart disease • Decreases clots in the bloodstream • Slows down development of arthritis • Slows the progression of diabetes-related complications	Pepper, garlic, broccoli, brussels sprouts, beef kidney, liver, Brazil nuts, chicken liver, egg yolks, mushrooms, tuna, wheat germ; whole grains are richer sources than refined flours
Sulforaphane	An antioxidant isothiocyanate	• Anti-cancer • Reduces risk of tobacco-induced tumors	Broccoli (30–50 times more concentrated in the immature broccoli sprouts), kale, radishes, cabbage, cauliflower, brussels sprouts, mustard greens
Vitamin A	Powerful antioxidant; fat-soluble (dissolves and can be stored in the body for long periods)	• Maintains healthy skin • Maintains healthy tissues in the mouth, digestive and urinary tracts, and genitals • Promotes reproductive development • Supports immune system • Anti-cancer	Sweet potatoes, carrots, melons

MICRO-NUTRIENT	WHAT IT IS	POTENTIAL HEALTH BENEFITS	WHERE IT'S FOUND
Vitamin C	Powerful antioxidant; water-soluble (moves through bloodstream quickly, so must be ingested regularly)	• Prevents scurvy • May fight the common cold • Helps maintain strong immune system • Helps prevent heart disease • Promotes healthy cholesterol levels • Anti-cancer • Strengthens collagen • Smokers need more	Most fruits, especially citrus, guavas, and papayas; tomatoes, green and red peppers, broccoli, spinach, potatoes, asparagus
Vitamin D	Powerful antioxidant; fat-soluble; found in food and can also be made in your body after exposure to ultraviolet rays from the sun; persons with darker skin require more since the high melanin content in their skin reduces the skin's ability to produce vitamin D from sunlight	• Maintains normal blood levels of calcium and phosphorus • Helps to form and maintain strong bones • Helps reduce osteoporosis and bone fracture, especially in post-menopausal women • Anti-cancer (especially colorectal)	Milk and other dairy products, cod liver oil, salmon, mackerel, tuna, sardines, eggs, beef liver, fortified foods
Vitamin E	Powerful antioxidant; fat-soluble	• Important in the formation of red blood cells • May be anti-cancer (especially prostate and breast, but conflicting reports) • May help prevent atherosclerosis • May help prevent blood clots that would lead to heart attacks • May reduce death from heart disease • May enhance immune function	Wheat germ, corn, nuts, seeds, olives, spinach and other green leafy vegetables, broccoli, asparagus, vegetable oils (corn, sunflower, soybean, cottonseed), kiwis, mangoes, avocadoes, fortified cereals

MICRO-NUTRIENT	WHAT IT IS	POTENTIAL HEALTH BENEFITS	WHERE IT'S FOUND
Vitamin K	Powerful antioxidant; fat-soluble	• Essential for normal blood clotting • Involved in bone formation and repair • May decrease the incidence or severity of osteoporosis and slow bone loss • Has been linked to increased longevity	Green leafy vegetables, spinach, broccoli, cabbage, cauliflower, asparagus, green tea, soybeans and soybean oil, cheese, liver, coffee, cereals

APPENDIX C

When It Comes to Fruits and Vegetables, Eat Colorfully!

IN NATURE, PLANTS OWE MANY OF THEIR BRIGHTEST COLORS TO A GROUP of over five hundred pigments called carotenoids. It is carotenoids that give plants, including fruits and vegetables, their yellow, orange, and red colors. Carotenoids are also present in green vegetables and plants, but their color is masked by green chlorophyll. Probably the best-known carotenoid is beta-carotene, which is found in many kinds of orange and yellow fruits and green leafy vegetables. As well as providing vitamin A, beta-carotene acts as an antioxidant. Lycopene is the pigment that gives tomatoes their bright red color. Lutein and zeaxanthin form the yellow of corn.

The more intensely colored a food is, the more disease-fighting properties it may have. For example, while white onions have been shown to boost the immune system, lower cholesterol, and protect against heart disease, red and yellow onions have even more nutrients. Furthermore, the more colors you are eating, the wider the range of nutrients you take in. So a good rule of thumb, when it comes to fruits and vegetables, is to eat as colorful a diet as possible!

COLOR	FRUIT AND VEGETABLE SOURCES	NUTRIENTS	WHAT THEY DO
White	Onion, garlic, chives, shallots, scallions, leeks	Allicin Indoles Sulforaphanes Polyphenols	May help fight cancer (especially prostate), lower cholesterol and blood pressure, and fight bodily infections
Green	Zucchini, broccoli, kale, cucumbers, honeydew melons, spinach, brussels sprouts, cabbage, cauliflower, watercress, asparagus, parsley, fresh dill, romaine lettuce, green peppers, avocadoes, peas	Vitamin K Beta-carotene Folate Lutein	Dark green foods are rich in antioxidants; beta-carotene is good for the eyes and reduces the risk of cancers and heart disease
Yellow	Squash, yellow peppers, corn	Beta-carotene Vitamin C Lutein Zeaxanthin	Some yellow vegetables, such as summer squash, contain the phytonutrient lutein, which helps protect against degeneration of eye structure with aging; zeaxanthin works along with lutein to maintain healthy eyes
Orange	Carrots, cantaloupes, pumpkins, sweet potatoes, peaches, nectarines, apricots, mangoes, oranges	Beta-carotene (converted to vitamin A in the body)	Anti-cancer benefits, may also prevent cataracts, slow the progression of heart disease, and boost the immune system
Red	Tomatoes, tomato sauce and paste, ketchup, watermelons, red grapefruit, red peppers	Lycopene Beta-carotene Vitamin C	Lycopene is an antioxidant that reduces the risk of prostate cancer and some other cancers, as well as cardiovascular disease

COLOR	FRUIT AND VEGETABLE SOURCES	NUTRIENTS	WHAT THEY DO
Red-Purple	Blueberries, cranberries, grapes and raisins, wine, cherries, plums and prunes, purple cabbage, strawberries, raspberries, eggplant, blackberries, figs	Anthocyanin	Powerful antioxidant that may help reduce risk of cancer, stroke, and heart disease; eating blueberries may benefit coordination and memory
Black-Dark Red	Black beans, kidney beans	Calcium Iron	Black beans are high in fiber and calcium; red beans are a good source of iron

APPENDIX D

Your Favorite Foods: Calories and Fats

FOOD	PORTION	FAT (G)	SAT. FAT (G)	CALORIES
FRUIT				
Apples	1 medium, skin on	.2	0	72
Apricots	3 medium	.1	0	50
Bananas	1 medium	.4	.1	105
Blueberries	1 cup	.5	0	83
Cantaloupe	1 cup cubes	.3	.1	54
Cherries, sweet red	½ cup	.1	0	37
Figs	2 dried	0	0	125
Grapefruit, pink or red	½ cup	.2	0	52
Grapes	1 cup	.3	.1	62
Honeydew	1 cup balls	.2	.1	64
Lemons	1	.3	0	22
Oranges	1medium	.2	0	62
Peaches	1 medium	.2	0	38
Pears	1 medium	.2	0	96
Pineapple	½ cup diced	.1	0	37
Plums	1medium	.2	0	30
Strawberries	1 cup halves	.5	0	49

FOOD	PORTION	FAT (G)	SAT. FAT (G)	CALORIES
Watermelon	1 cup balls	.2	0	46
Apple juice	1 cup	.3	0	117
Lemon juice	Juice from 1 lemon	0	0	12
Orange juice	1 cup	.5	0	112
Pineapple juice	1 cup	.2	0	140
Prune juice	1 cup	.1	0	182
VEGETABLES				
Artichoke	1	5	0	150
Asparagus	1 medium spear	0	0	3
Broccoli	½ cup	0	0	22
Carrots	½ cup	0	0	35
Cauliflower	½ cup	0	0	14
Celery	½ cup	0	0	5
Corn	½ cup	.9	.1	66
Cucumber	½ cup	.1	0	8
Eggplant	½ cup	.1	0	10
Garlic	1 clove	0	0	4
Green beans	1 cup	.1	0	34
Iceberg lettuce	1 cup	.1	0	6
Mushrooms	1 cup	.2	0	15
Onions	½ cup	0	0	33
Peppers, red bell	½ cup	.2	.1	20
Potatoes	½ cup	.1	0	29
Pumpkin	½ cup	.1	0	15
Spinach	1 cup	.1	0	7
Squash, summer	½ cup	.1	0	9
Tomatoes, cherry	½ cup	.1	0	7
Zucchini	½ cup	.1	0	10
LEGUMES				
Black beans	½ cup cooked	.5	.1	114
Chickpeas, canned	½ cup	1.3	.2	143
Fava beans	½ cup cooked	.3	<.1	93
Great northern beans	½ cup cooked	.4	.1	104
Hummus	½ cup	10.6	1.4	218
Kidney beans, canned	½ cup	.4	<.1	104
Lentils	½ cup cooked	.4	<.1	115
Lima beans, canned	½ cup	.2	<.1	95
Navy beans	½ cup cooked	.5	.2	127

FOOD	PORTION	FAT (G)	SAT. FAT (G)	CALORIES
Peas, green, frozen	½ cup boiled	.2	0	62
Peas, split	½ cup boiled	.4	<.1	115
Pink beans	½ cup cooked	.4	.1	126
Pinto beans	½ cup cooked	.4	.1	117
Cannellini beans, canned	½ cup	.4	.1	153
NUTS AND SEEDS				
Almonds	1 oz	9	.7	103
Hazelnuts	1 oz	10.3	.8	106
Peanuts	1 oz	8.8	1.2	102
Pumpkin	1 oz	7.9	1.5	93
Sunflower	1 oz	2.85	.3	26
Walnuts	1 oz	8.2	.9	82
GRAINS				
Bread, pita, white	1 large	.7	.1	165
Bread, white	1 slice	1.0	.2	80
Bread, whole-wheat	1 slice	1.2	.3	69
Macaroni, white	½ cup cooked	.5	<.1	99
Macaroni, whole-wheat	½ cup cooked	.4	<.1	85
Rice, brown	½ cup cooked	.9	.2	108
Rice, white	½ cup cooked	.2	<.1	103
Barley	½ cup cooked	.4	<.1	95
Buckwheat	½ cup cooked	.5	.1	78
Oats	½ cup cooked	1.2	.2	74
Wheat flour	½ cup	.6	.1	227
Cornflakes	½ cup	.1	<.1	50
DAIRY				
Cheese, American	1.5 oz	10.5	6.4	127
Cheese, blue	1.5 oz	12.1	8	150
Cheese, cheddar	1.5 oz	14.1	9	171
Cheese, cream	1.5 oz	14.8	9.2	149
Cheese, feta	1.5 oz	9	6.3	110
Cheese, mozzarella	1.5 oz	9.4	5.5	127
Cheese, parmesan	1 Tbsp grated	1.4	.9	22
Cheese, swiss	1 oz	7.9	5.0	108

FOOD	PORTION	FAT (G)	SAT. FAT (G)	CALORIES
Cottage cheese, 2%	1 cup	4.4	2.8	203
Egg Beaters	¼ cup	0	0	30
Eggs	1 whole	10.2	3.1	148
Milk, 1%	1 cup	2.4	1.5	102
Milk, skim	1 cup	.6	0	91
Yogurt, low-fat, plain	8 oz	4	2.5	155
Yogurt, fat-free, plain	8 oz	0	0	135
Yogurt, low-fat, fruit	8 oz	2	1.3	240
Yogurt, fat-free, sugar-free, fruit	8 oz	0	0	120
MEAT				
Chicken, ground	3 oz raw	7.5	2.3	68
Chicken breast	3 oz raw	1.2	0	90
Lamb chop	3 oz raw	26.3	11.3	293
Pork chop	3 oz raw	4.5	1.5	120
Turkey, ground	3 oz raw	.4	0	98
Turkey breast	2 slices	.6	.2	41
Veal cutlet	3 oz raw	22.5	0	293
SEAFOOD				
Clams	3 oz cooked	.8	.1	63
Cod	3 oz cooked	.7	.1	89
Halibut	3 oz cooked	2.5	.3	118
Lobster	3 oz cooked	.5	.1	83
Mackerel	3 oz cooked	15.1	3.5	223
Mussels	3 oz cooked	.9	.2	84
Salmon	3 oz cooked	3.8	.6	127
Shrimp	3 oz cooked	.9	.2	84
Snapper	3 oz cooked	1.5	.3	109
Tilefish	3 oz cooked	4.0	.7	125
Tuna	3 oz cooked	1.0	.3	118
Tuna, canned	3 oz	.7	.2	99
Whitefish	3 oz cooked	6.4	1.0	146
OIL				
Canola	2 Tbsp	18	2	240
Corn	2 Tbsp	27.2	3.4	240
Olive	2 Tbsp	27	3.6	240
Peanut	2 Tbsp	27	4.6	240
Sesame	2 Tbsp	27.2	3.8	240
Soybean	2 Tbsp	27.2	4	240
Sunflower	2 Tbsp	27.2	3.6	240
Vegetable, (usually all or mostly soybean oil)	2 Tbsp	27.2	3.4	240
Walnut	2 Tbsp	27.2	2.4	240
WINE				
Wine, red	4 oz	0	0	85
Wine, white	4 oz	0	0	80

Index

About the Authors

Angelo Acquista, M.D., received his medical degree at New York University School of Medicine in 1981 and is affiliated with Lenox Hill Hospital in Manhattan as an attending physician and clinical instructor in the Intensive Care Unit. He is board-certified in internal medicine, pulmonary medicine, and tropical diseases. He is an Honorary Police Surgeon of the New York City Police Department. Dr. Acquista has had a keen interest in nutrition and fitness for many years, both personally and on behalf of his patients.

Laurie A. Vandermolen received a B.A. from the University of Michigan and attended the Hunter College Graduate School of Biological Sciences. She has been a medical writer at academic medical institutions for over ten years. Her positions included a post at Rockefeller University, where she studied the behavior and metabolism of lean and obesity-prone rodents on various diets. She lives in New York City with her husband.

About the Type

This book was set in Goudy, a typeface designed by Frederic William Goudy (1865–1947). Goudy began his career as a bookkeeper, but devoted the rest of his life to the pursuit of "recognized quality" in a printing type.

Goudy was produced in 1914 and was an instant bestseller for the foundry. It has generous curves and smooth, even color. It is regarded as one of Goudy's finest achievements.